BRAND POSITIONING IN PHARMA

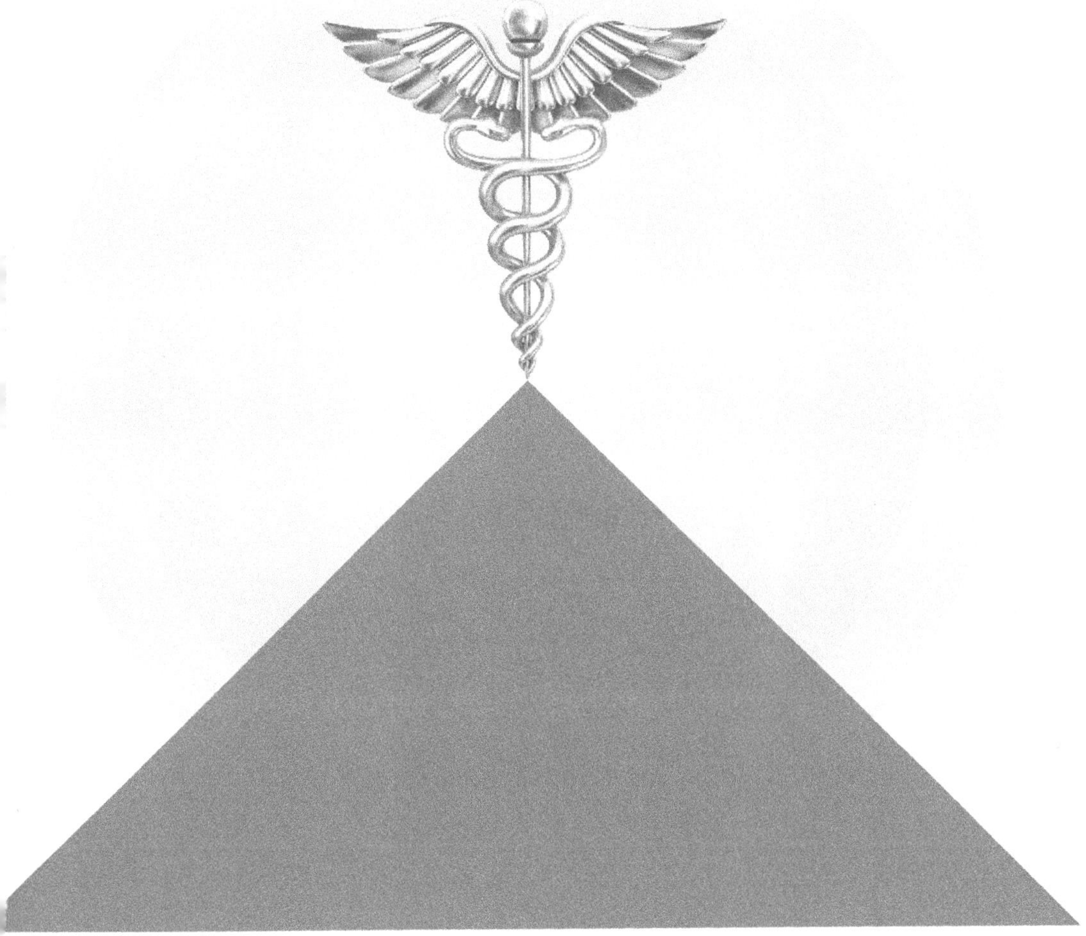

BRAND POSITIONING IN PHARMA

Subba Rao Chaganti

PharmaMed Press
An imprint of BSP Books Pvt. Ltd.
4-4-309/316, Giriraj Lane,
Sultan Bazar, Hyderabad - 500 095.

Brand Positioning in Pharma
by *Subba Rao Chaganti*

Published by

PharmaMed Press
An imprint of BSP Books Pvt. Ltd.
4-4-309/316, Giriraj Lane, Sultan Bazar, Hyderabad - 500 095.
Phone: 040-23445688, 23445600; Fax: 91+40-23445611
E-mail: info@pharmamedpress.com
www.pharmamedpress.com/pharmamedpress.net

Cover Design

J. Siva Prasad, Amita Designs

ISBN: 978-93-95039-51-2 (Hardbound)

Dedicated to the late Professor Tarun Gupta
(December 27, 1939, to October 31, 2017)

The legendary marketing guru who transformed marketing in the Indian pharmaceutical industry since 1970. He introduced the ubiquitous visual aid and many marketing concepts, strategies, and practices that are still relevant and valid even today.

ACKNOWLEDGEMENTS

I thank the late Prof. Tarun Gupta, who introduced and taught me everything I needed to know about positioning as early as 1978. Since then, the body of knowledge about positioning has grown significantly with contributions from various marketing scholars and practitioners. Therefore, I must thank every one of them for their significant contributions to expanding our understanding of positioning and how to apply them to build brands of products, services, and even businesses.

I must express my gratitude to all those who have helped me in this long journey of fifty-five years in pharmaceutical marketing. But, unfortunately, there are far too many of them to mention here. My sincere thanks to all my teachers, peers, colleagues, and students who have helped me widen my horizon and broaden my perspectives on marketing in general and pharmaceutical marketing in particular.

A few individuals' help and support have been truly significant in bringing about this book, Brand Positioning in Pharma. Without their physical, intellectual, and moral support, this book would still be in the conceptual stage. I sincerely thank:

- Mr. J. Sivaprasad, managing director of Amita Designs, for designing a fantastic cover for the book
- Anil Shah the most enthusiastic publisher with a passion for publishing that I have known
- Nikunjesh Shah for making the digital versions of this book available
- Mr. Naresh Daver and his team and Pharma Med Press for designing this book beautifully

Last but not least, I owe my thanks to Mahalakshmi, my better half, both literally and figuratively, for supporting me throughout the writing of this book. I must also thank my three children and their spouses—Srinivasa Phanindra, Geetha, Lavanya, Aditya, Soumya, and Chaitanya for their appreciation and feedback during this book project. In addition, my son, Srinivasa Phanindra, has been very encouraging with his constructive feedback on the initial draft of this book.

More importantly, I thank my grandchildren— Aditi, Eesha, Surya, and Shriya. They have been a constant source of joy, happiness, and inspiration that contributed greatly to the writing of this book. The sparkle in their eyes when they saw their names as I wrote them in acknowledgements gave me immense satisfaction.

PROLOGUE

I learned about the positioning concept in marketing in a product management workshop in February 1978 conducted by the late Prof. Tarun Gupta, a legendary marketing professional heading Glaxo Pharma in India. He gave the participants a reprint of the original article, The Positioning Era Cometh, written by the pioneers of positioning, Jack Trout and Al Ries, and published in the Advertising Age as an essential reading before the workshop. He was a great teacher with an uncanny knack for making complex topics simple and easy to understand. I have been hooked on the positioning concept since I attended that workshop on positioning in the Indian pharmaceutical industry. It was the first-ever workshop on positioning in the pharmaceutical industry in India, and Glaxo was the first-ever company to apply positioning strategies to promote its products.

Later, I continued to study the theory and practice of positioning, grabbing every article, literature, and book that dealt with positioning. I also tried applying the positioning concepts to every brand I managed over the years, differentiating them in every way I could.

This book, Brand Positioning in Pharma, is an effort to share all my learnings with all the practicing and aspiring pharma brand managers to help them differentiate their brands so they can win in the marketplace.

The book has six chapters— Brand Positioning, Disease Branding, Drug Repurposing and Repositioning, Blue Ocean Strategy, Framing, and Brand Positioning in the Digital Age. While the first three chapters and the fifth chapter are about product positioning, one may ask what chapters like Framing and Blue Ocean Strategy are doing in a book on Positioning.

When you think of it, Framing and Blue Ocean strategy have the concept of differentiation at their core, just like Positioning does. However, in the case of the Blue Ocean Strategy, the source of differentiation is value-based innovation.

At the same time, Framing is how a company tries to create an impression or image of the product in the consumers' mind by specifying or changing a frame of reference. Here lies the difference between Framing and Positioning. In the case of Positioning, you do it by tweaking the 4 Ps (Product, Place, Promotion, and Price) to create the differentiation, but in Framing, one reframes by changing the frame of reference.

Thus, Framing and Blue Ocean Strategy are closely related to Positioning concepts essentially to differentiate a company's products and services to win in the hyper-competitive marketplace.

I tried to address all aspects of positioning to answer vital questions such as the *What*, *Why*, and *How* of positioning. I have also compiled about fifty-two cases to illustrate how brand managers in pharma have applied different positioning concepts to make their brands stand out in a crowd and become leaders in their categories. I believe these cases will facilitate experiential learning and ignite creative sparks necessary to differentiate their brands in today's me-too world and the age of sameness.

I believe you will find reading this book as illuminating and enjoyable as I felt while writing it.

Hyderabad **Subba Rao Chaganti**
November 5, 2022

CONTENTS

Cases:

CHAPTER 3

Drug Repositioning by Repurposing Drugs, Drug Repositioning: Two Approaches, Experiment-based Approach, In Silico-based Approach, Two Main Strategies, On-target Drug Repurposing, Off-target Drug Repurposing, Big Opportunity

Cases:

LIST OF ABBREVIATIONS

AD	Alzheimer's Disease
AAP	American Academy of Pediatrics
ADD	Attention Deficit Disorder
ADHD	Attention Deficit Hyperactivity Disorder
ACS	Acute Coronary Syndrome
AIDS	Acquired Immunodeficiency Syndrome
ALL	Acute Lymphocytic Leukemia
AML	Acute Myeloid Leukemia
ALCL	Ana-plastic Large Cell Lymphoma
APA	American Psychiatric Association
ARB	Angiotensin Receptor Blocker
CCB	Calcium Channel Blocker
CML	Chronic Myelogenous Leukemia
CVD	Cardio Vascular Disease
DSM	Diagnostic and Statistical Manual of Mental Disorders
DTC	Direct-to-Consumer
DTCA	Direct-to-Consumer-Advertising
ED	Erectile Dysfunction
FDA	Food and Drug Administration
GERD	Gastroesophageal Reflux Disease
GIDH	Glaxo Institute for Digestive Health
GIST	Gastrointestinal Stromal Tumor
HIV	Human Immunodeficiency Virus
ICS	International Continence Society
IBD	Inflammatory Bowel Disease
KOL	Key Opinion Leader
MIT	Massachusetts Institute of Technology
MS	Multiple Sclerosis
MSD	Merck Sharp and Dohme
NCE	New Chemical Entity
NDA	New Drug Application
NIH	National Institutes of Health

NIMH	National Institutes of Mental Health
NSAID	Non-Steroidal Anti-inflammatory Drug
NSCLC	Non-small Cell Lung Cancer
OAB	Overactive Bladder
OCD	Obsessive-Compulsive Disorder
PDAC	Psycho Pharmacological Drug Advisory Committee
PCP	Primary Care Physician
PDE	Phosphodiesterase
PMS	Premenstrual Syndrome
PMDD	Premenstrual Dysphoric Disorder
PMRG	Pharmaceutical Marketing Research Group
POD	Points of Difference
POM	Prescription-only Medicine
POP	Points of Parity
PTSD	Post-Traumatic Stress Disorder
RA	Rheumatoid Arthritis
RCC	Renal Cell Carcinoma
RLS	Restless Leg Syndrome
SAD	Social Anxiety Disorder
SSRI	Selective Serotonin Reuptake Inhibitor
TKI	Tyrosine Kinase Inhibitor
TRD	Treatment-Resistant Depression
USP	Unique Selling Proposition

CHAPTER

1

Brand Positioning

Today's marketplace is no longer responsive to the advertising that worked in the past. There are just too many products, too many companies, and too much marketing noise. To succeed in our over-communicated society, a company must create a position in the prospect's mind. A position that considers not only its strength and weaknesses but also those of its competitors.

– Jack Trout and Al Ries, in their article, The Positioning Era Cometh, The Advertising Age, April 24, 1972

Jack Trout and Al Ries coined the word Positioning. They mentioned it for the first time in their 1969 article titled *Positioning is the game people play in today's me-too marketplace* in Industrial Marketing.

In 1971, David Ogilvy, one of the founding fathers of modern advertising, pointed out that our campaigns' results depend less on how we write our advertising than on how a product is positioned. Thus, the 1970s ushered in a new era in marketing— The Era of Positioning. Accurate Positioning has become the most important step in effective marketing.

Later, the positioning pioneers Jack Trout and Al Ries wrote a highly influential article highlighting the positioning concept, *The Positioning Era Cometh* in the Advertising Age, on April 24, 1972. They wrote:

Today's marketplace is no longer responsive to the advertising that worked in the past. There are just too many products, too many companies, and too much marketing noise. To succeed in our over-communicated society, a company must create a position in the prospect's mind. A position that considers not only its strength and weaknesses but also those of its competitors.

A few years later, in 1981, they published the first book on Positioning, *Positioning: The Battle for your mind*, which sold over three million copies worldwide.

Evolution of the Positioning Concept

1. **USP (Unique Selling Proposition)** concept popularized by Rosser Reeves originated in the '40s. However, USP did not consider the competition.
2. **The next big Idea:** David Ogilvy's Brand Image as opposed to the actual product difference (as in the USP), came later.
3. Jack Trout and Al Ries came up with the next big idea of **Brand Perception and Positioning**, taking marketing to the next level in the late '60s.

It's All About Perception!

Marco De Veglia wrote about an interview he had with Jack Trout recently in his book, *Brand Positioning Formula*. So, here is the latest take of Jack Trout on positioning according to that interview: *The world was getting more competitive, and in the world of competition, it is all about perception. You win or lose in the mind of your prospect, building perceptions. So, it is not a question of reality as much as perception. And that makes perception a reality that makes marketing more of a perception game. So, that is how the concept of positioning your brand in the customer's mind is born*.

So, Positioning is the process of establishing a product, person, event, company, or even an object in the minds of the members of a target market in such a way that it is perceived to answer the needs of that market better than the competition does. Positioning thus refers to the identification and communication of a differential advantage.

Profitable Positioning is a strategy for creating a unique product image, which increases total profits. Firms planning modifications of existing products or introducing new products will naturally, in keeping with their marketing objectives, strive to position their products' entry to produce maximum sales and profits.

Product positioning is a concept borrowed from military strategy. We can find the earliest known writings about positioning in military strategy in the writings of a Chinese general, Sun Tzu, a contemporary of Confucius, the famous Chinese philosopher. In his classic work, *The art of War*, Sun Tzu, the master strategist he was, discussed the importance of positioning in the military strategy context— *troop disposition, ground, terrain, relative strength of opposing forces, and the mental attitudes of the opposition. His primary target was the mind of the opposing commander*. These concepts are very much relevant in the present-day marketing context.

What is A Brand?

Before we get to how to position a brand in the minds of consumers, let us have a common definition of what a brand is, as there are many definitions of what a brand is. Four experts define brands as :

1. A brand is the intangible sum of a product's attributes. (David Ogilvy)

2. A brand is the set of assets and liabilities linked to a brand's name and symbol that adds or subtracts from the value a product or service provides to a firm or that firm's customer. (David Aaker)
3. A brand is a set of expectations, memories, and relationships that are taken together to choose one product or service over another. (Seth Godin)
4. Your brand is what other people say about you when you are not in the room. (Jeff Bezos)

While all these are great definitions from experts in the field, they are not actionable. They do not tell you how to create a brand. So, here is a more actionable definition: *A brand is the sum of all associations consumers have about your offering. Those associations form the brand image, which, together with the brand's awareness (unaided) levels, form your brand's equity.*

Brand Associations

How do you know what associations consumers have with your brand? First, ask them what comes to mind when they think of your brand and you have your brand associations.

Brand associations are images and symbols associated with a brand or a brand benefit. At the same time, brand associations are not reasons-to-buy but can create a differentiation based on a brand's perceived qualities that are not replicable. Brand associations are the attributes that come to the consumer's mind when discussing the brand. They help consumers recognize the brand within its category because the consumer relates the brand's association to the explicit and implicit meanings. Here are some factors that help form brand associations:

- Customers coming into contact with the organization, its products, and employees
- Word-of-mouth publicity
- Quality of the product
- Advertisements
- Product class or category to which the brand belongs

- Price at which the brand is sold
- Celebrity endorsements

Consumers develop positive brand associations if their experiences are positive with brand communication and the values that the brand stands for align with theirs.

Since brand associations are the thoughts that enter a consumer's mind when they think about a brand, marketers are continuously striving to create a mental connection a consumer makes between a brand and some other factor, such as a concept, person, interest, experience, emotion, activity, or image.

Consumers will automatically form associations with your brand, whether you want that association or not, and whether you manage them. Consumers will automatically put your brand into mental categories and associate specific meanings with it based on their experiences, knowledge, belief systems, values, and what they hear from others (word of mouth), including their friends, family, peers, or the media. Therefore, you must proactively create positive associations for your brand to differentiate it so it can stand out from the crowd.

How to create a favorable and memorable brand association? The three fundamental elements of building brand associations are visuals, language, and personification.

Brand Personification

Brand personification is a projective technique where you ask people to think about brands as if they were people and to describe how the brands would think and feel. You start this process by exploring your brand's personality traits. The key questions to ask and answer are:

- For example, if your *brand* were a person, not a product or service, would *it* be a man or woman?
- Street-smart or book-smart?
- Extrovert or introvert?

- What would be the age of that person (brand)? Young? Middle-aged or old?
- Would the person (brand) be caring and understanding or tough and authoritative?
- Also, you can think of your brand as a person, a celebrity, or a role model who best characterizes your brand's attributes and features.

Here is a case highlighting the importance of brand personification, where researchers surveyed physicians to understand the brand personality of a prescription drug.

CASE

1

How Do You Personify A Brand?!

When using this tool, the moderator asks questions that project a human aura onto your product, such as,'where was drug x born? Where did it go to school? What kind of books and sports does drug X like? While it may sound odd, personification yields unexpected responses that allow you to see how people perceive a product.

For example, researchers asked respondents about a leading drug for treating acute coronary syndrome (ACS). In response to a question about where physicians thought the drug had attended college, several respondents suggested MIT (Massachusetts Institute of Technology)— making the marketer aware that the product was perceived as technically sophisticated. Understanding this allowed the marketing to build a successful positioning strategy incorporating the concept.

Creating a brand personality and character will help you present your brand in human form, enabling strong associations in the customers' minds and reinforcing the positive perception.

Brand Positioning

Philip Kotler, the marketing guru, defined brand positioning as designing the company's offering and image to occupy a distinctive place in the target market's mind. In other words, brand positioning describes how a brand differs from its competitors and where or how it sits in the customers' minds. Therefore, brand positioning is just how you differentiate your product or company in the customer's mind.

Acknowledging the contribution of the positioning pioneers, Philip Kotler said there is a step that shall precede the 4 Ps of marketing. That step is another **P** for Positioning, the revolutionary concept that Jack Trout and Al Ries introduced in their book on Positioning. So, Positioning must precede all marketing activities. For example, brand marketing starts with Positioning, putting your brand in the customer's mind differently from competitors, making it more interesting for your target audience.

Brand Positioning in Pharma

Why is Positioning a Must?

It is the information explosion that has led to this realization. The ever-increasing noise level in the marketplace, with the number of brands multiplying like rabbits, has made positioning a *Must* for survival and growth. For example, let us consider the pharmaceutical industry in India. Over 10,000 companies are churning out over 100,000 products. An urban doctor meets about 20 to 25 medical representatives on a typical working day who detail about 5 to 8 products. That means exposure to anything between 100 to 200 products. Add to this the information through newspapers, magazines, professional journals, radio and television messages, etc. The Total number of messages that he is exposed to, is truly mind-blogging. A marketer must virtually fight for the doctor's attention for his product. While the human mind can cope with such an information overload, how it deals with and processes this excessive volume of information is certainly not helpful to the marketer. One is the screening and selective process of perception. The other is that the human mind rejects information unrelated to prior knowledge. The human mind has no room for something new unless it is in some way related to or matches with prior information and knowledge. The simplest example is that learning the alphabet of any language is essential for learning words in that language. Without prior knowledge of the alphabet, new words sound like gibberish.

Furthermore, it is said that people rank objects, events, and even other people in their minds. It is necessary to organize the ever-increasing information to cope with it. Therefore, consumers rank products in their minds. If the product is distinctly different in that product category and fits with a similar, equivalent perception of the consumer, only then is the product likely to be ranked higher in the consumer's mind. The closer and more perfect the unique product attribute and the consumer perception fit, the higher the ranking of that product. It is here that the Positioning of the product is going to play a vital, crucial role. Much depends on how the product is positioned.

Positioning Prescription Drug Brands

Brand positioning is about the customer, not the brand, so it is customer-driven. It involves identifying the target group's current needs, addressing those, and offering compelling reasons to choose the brand over competitors. The way to achieve this is to define product attributes (in the case of in-market brands) and design (in the case of new products) product attributes that are relevant to customers, which competition does not have, and communicate them effectively.

Since brand positioning is customer-driven, you must ensure that the customer plays an active role in developing your brand positioning to understand their needs and to make your brand more relevant. Therefore, brand positioning is the first step in developing and building a brand preceding all other marketing activities. Also, almost all strategic activities depend on clear, precise brand positioning.

A Different Ball Game

While there are many similarities in marketing CPG (Consumer Packaged Goods) and prescription drugs, significant differences, too, exist. Consider these, for example:

- Pharmaceutical brands have patents that expire about ten to twelve years from launch, with research and development costing about $2.6 billion per drug.
- A very low success rate of 1 in 10,000 drugs screened for development.
- People *want* to buy CPG brands to express their aspirations, whereas they do not seek to buy a healthcare product but do so because they *need* to.

These differences apart, all positioning principles apply to prescription drug brands too. However, before we get to the positioning process of pharma brands, we need to understand thoroughly:

- The marketing environment in which your brand will compete
- The target market, including relevant trends in your category and disease state, by applying outside-in thinking, which means standing in the customer's shoes and viewing everything the company does through the customer's eyes.
- Feeling things from their perspective, walking in their shoes, spending a day in their life, and seeing how they see them to gain customer insights. Therefore, it is important to uncover their needs, wants, frustrations and pain points better than competitors.
- Compete by analyzing competitors thoroughly. As Sun Tzu, the Chinese General and military strategist, said, you need to understand your enemy intimately to beat them. Therefore, it would be great once you determine who your core competitors are, if you become them, stepping into their shoes so that you can deeply understand them. In other words, you should practice competitive simulation.
- Above all, you should understand your brand thoroughly inside out. You must understand the product attributes, strengths, weaknesses, brand perceptions, brand image, emotional and experiential associations, and how they align with the customer's needs and wants and address their pain points.

Once you develop a deep understanding of the marketing environment, your target market, customers, and competition, it is time to do a complete competitive SWOT (Strengths, Weaknesses, Opportunities, Threats) analysis so that you can identify points of parity and points of differentiation and create a winning positioning strategy.

Understanding the Marketing Environment

Usually, pharma marketers will have an informed opinion about the market, brand, and opportunity based on a quick, early, and knowledge-based assessment and may not have done the rigorous due diligence required to understand the environment, customer, and competition thoroughly. The marketing team would have obtained the customer insights from their KOLs (Key Opinion

Leaders). However, while KOLs are important stakeholders with relevant expertise in their specialty areas having valid perspectives, they often do not reflect the real world because they are not in the trenches treating patients daily, handling access issues, and managing the patient problems the average clinician encounters daily. As a result, companies do not completely understand the marketplace and fail to develop the market, educate prescribers and patients or convince payers. That internal product-centric approach may be one of the major reasons why more pharma brands fail. They need to ask questions like:

- How are your customers changing?
- How are their needs evolving, and how are they solving them?
- What are the competitors' moves?
- Are there innovators entering the market that will transform or disrupt it?

It would help you significantly if you focused on trends most relevant to your customers, the disease and therapy areas, and your brand. For example, your analysis can focus on the following:

- *Health factor*s: demographics, culture, aging, obesity, language, exercise, smoking, drug use and addiction, social determinants of health (SDoH)—income, food, housing, transportation, etc.
- *Healthcare system*: Changes in policy, universal policy, universal healthcare coverage, underserved populations, Medicare, Medicaid, regulations, Food and Drug Administration (FDA) policy, uninsured, overinsured patient populations
- *Healthcare industry*: vertical integration, consolidations, insurance reform, scientific innovation, precision medicine, genetics, research and development, services
- *Other trend*s include increasing consumerism in healthcare, health literacy, care anywhere, technological advancements, including wearables, telehealth, and value-based care, and how they affect healthcare.

Monitoring these changing trends will help you understand their impact on several things that affect your performance, such as changes in public policies, regulations, and government agencies; access to physicians, hospitals, and payers; and delivery of care to patients leading to improved patient outcomes.

Understanding the Target Market

What your market is may look like a very simple question, but it is a deceptively simple one. You must dive deep into its many layers to understand the market segment effectively and uncover the opportunities.

The dictionary defines the term market as the total of all the buyers and sellers in the area or regions under consideration. This definition implies that the market is more about buyers and sellers than the products. On further analysis, it is about the value sought by the buyer and provided by the seller, which means the market is more about customers than products. So, we must define the market from the customer's point of view or in a customer-centric way.

Brian Smith emphasizes this point in his book *Brand Therapy*. *You can't create a strong brand strategy until you really understand your market, and you can't understand your market until you define it the same way as your customer does*.

Traditionally, pharmaceutical companies have a product-centric view of the market and developed a strong product-oriented culture. So, they define their market in product terms. For example, market data usually defines the market size as the aggregate of all the products sold in that market. Competitors are defined as other firms that make the same product type. And customers are those who currently buy from competitors or us. However, this product-based definition of the market has some major disadvantages. Consider these for example:

- In most pharma markets, product usage and the market for the products are very different things. For example, think of the number of untreated patients with mental illness, where competition may not be a similar product but therapies such as counseling.

- In addition, the product-oriented market definition tends to focus on healthcare professionals, when payers and patients increasingly play an important part in their healthcare decision-making.

Assessing Market Opportunity: Potential or Actual?

Assume that you want to introduce a non-steroidal anti-inflammatory drug. What should you consider as your market? Your *actual* (directly competing market) would mean an aggregate sales volume of all non-steroidal anti-inflammatory drugs. That is limiting the market and restricting opportunities.

Looking at the *potential* market would mean widening the horizon of opportunities. The potential market, in this case, would be the *anti-arthritic market* as a whole since NSAIDs are widely used in the treatment of arthritis due to their safety and efficacy. When you analyze doctors' prescriptions, you will observe that the anti-arthritic market includes, in addition to NSAIDs, muscle relaxants, steroids, topical rubifacients, anti-gout preparations, analgesics, etc. With the help of prescription audit report figures, it is possible to quantify the size of each segment. You can find exactly how many prescriptions are written for every competing product in each segment.

Consider, for example, the gout segment of the anti-arthritic market. The prescriptions written for gout include, apart from the anti-gout preparations like Zyloric (Burroughs Wellcome then and GSK now) and Benemid (Merind then and MSD now), NSAIDs (Non-steroidal Anti-inflammatory Drugs) and analgesics. By referring to the prescription audit, you can find out the exact number of prescriptions written for NSAIDs in gout;

- Prescriptions written for analgesics in gout
- In addition, the total number of prescriptions written for the more specific anti-gout preparations

Armed with this ammunition of information, you can now aim to be going great guns with your new NSAID against a bigger anti-arthritic market (potential market) rather than confirming yourself to a smaller NSAID market (actual market).

Similarly, when you analyze each of the major segments like pain, lumbago, sciatica, bursitis, synovitis, spondylitis, sprains, osteoarthritis, rheumatic arthritis, etc, (based on diagnostic profile), you would observe that the *actual market* of NSAIDS allows itself to expand into a much larger *potential (anti-arthritic) market!*

You can do a similar analysis taking into account all the aspects of exploring and evaluating new opportunities in all the markets you want to enter. The following case shows how defining your potential market can help your brand succeed.

CASE

2

What's Your Market? Clear Market Definition Makes Revital A Mega Brand!

What is Your Market?

What is your market? Simple as it may seem, it is one of the most important strategic questions. When entering an existing market, what do you consider your market as? The total of direct competitors and their combined market share? Or do you also consider indirect competition in defining your market?

The Case of Revital

The year was 1988. The market comprised revitalizers, a group of all ginseng-containing formulations. ORG (Operations Research Group) grouped all ginseng-containing preparations into Rejuvenators. Four companies participated in this new segment in 1988— Duphar Interfran (now Solvay), Micro Labs, Alembic, and Biological E. Limited was a new entrant with a different version - Korean Red Ginseng, which was supposed to be a superior variety of ginseng. The total Revitalizer market containing ginseng preparations was around ₹ 100 million. All these current players have defined their market as ginseng-containing preparations and aimed at about ten percent market share. Consequently, their promotional effort was limited by their vision of their market definition.

At the same time, Ranbaxy was planning to enter the Rejuvenators market. After doing the market opportunity analysis, the company formulated ginseng differently. Around the same time, Pharmaton, a Switzerland-based pharmaceutical company, was marketing a formulation that contained ginseng and b-complex factors. Ranbaxy spotted an opportunity to differentiate its ginseng formulation and developed a formulation containing ginseng, b-complex factors, and several other multivitamin and minerals. They realized that the market opportunity of the b-complex vitamins and minerals market is ten-times bigger than the rejuvenators market, at ₹ 1 billion as compared to ₹ 100 million of the Rejuvenators market. The company named the new formulation, *Revital* very appropriately and positioned it as a b-complex vitamin-mineral supplement with a huge difference, containing ginseng, the rejuvenator. They set a marketing objective of ₹ 100 million in the launch year, which is the same size as the total rejuvenators market. The company planned an aggressive marketing strategy, invested appropriately, and rallied the whole company behind it. The rest is history. Ranbaxy became a blockbuster in the launch year and became a mega brand.

The case of Revital is a classic case of what a proper market definition can do to your brand strategy and make it a huge success!

Understanding Your Customers

Before we begin understanding the customers, let's define *the customer*. In healthcare, there is no single customer, and the term *customer* includes doctors, nurses, payers, patients, and caregivers of patients. At the same time, we use the word *consumers* to refer to patients, caregivers, and their families, as they are the end users of products and services. Consumers are still customers, but they are the end users of our products and not typically healthcare professionals who make prescribing decisions on behalf of patients (consumers). So, consumers refer to only patients or caregivers, while customers refer to patients, caregivers, HCPs, payers, and other stakeholders.

The main purpose of understanding the stakeholders is to gain customer insights by uncovering their needs, wants, and pain points so you can address them better than your competitors. What is *insight*? It is a deep-seated need from the customer's perspective, unlocking an opportunity to inspire customer action and win in the market.

The process of gaining customer insights involves stakeholder analysis, segmentation and targeting, patient journey, and identifying the moments of truth.

Stakeholder Analysis

In healthcare marketing, the main stakeholders are the patient (consumer), the doctor (prescriber), and the insurer (payer). Some disease states could also have the caregiver (consumer), nurses, clinic staff, support groups, and health coaches as stakeholders. While the patient and the doctor are the key stakeholders in every disease, the question of which of the two is the key decision-maker depends on many factors like the disease, the healthcare system, culture, education, and income. The disease state plays a major role in determining the *weightage* given to the influence of the patient or the doctor. For example, a cancer patient's insights are extremely important in oncology. At the same time, the oncologist's role assumes even greater importance, considering the complexity and urgency of care and innovative science. So, the oncologist becomes the key decision-maker.

On the other hand, in the case of erectile dysfunction (ED), the educated patient may ask the doctor for the medication by name (Cialis or Viagra), avoiding the awkward discussion regarding symptoms. In such cases, the prescribing doctor is completely out of the decision-making process, and the patient becomes a true consumer making a decision. Therefore, stakeholders' relative importance is useful when deciding your brand positioning.

Segmentation and Targeting

Segmentation is the process of separating the defined market into customer groups with similar characteristics, needs, attitudes, behaviors, and choice drivers, who form the market. While you need to segment HCPs, patients, and other stakeholders to mine their insights, brand positioning should focus on patient insights. This is because patient insights are important to HCPs, too, to treat their conditions effectively.

Key Questions

Here are a few key questions to be answered while segmenting your market. They will help you sharpen the focus.

1. **What has been the basis for segmentation?**
   - Demographic
   - Geographical
   - Age Group
   - Gender
   - Income levels
   - Therapeutic Group – By nature of the disease
   - The severity of the disease – Acute, chronic, recurrent, recalcitrant
   - The therapeutic benefits your products offer distinctly
   - Usage rate

- The place of treatment – Home (GP), Nursing Home, Government Hospital, or Primary
- Health Centre – Private Hospital – Corporate Hospital
- The specialty of the doctor – Gynecologist, dermatologist, cardiologist, etc.

2. **Questions related to customers and consumers while segmenting the market:**
   1. What are the needs of consumers (patients)?
   2. What are the needs of intermediate customers (doctors who are influencers)?
   3. Are there any natural relationships between the consumers and the customers in the segment?
   - Do old patients consult old doctors?
   - Do women patients go to lady doctors?
   - Do the highly educated, upper-income patients go to specialists and super specialists?
3. **Questions related to the viability of segments:**
   - Are the segments attractive enough?
   - Do they have adequate sales potential?
   - Are they growing rapidly enough?
   - Are they crowded with the competition?
   - Can they support your promotional costs and earn adequate returns or profits?

HCP Segmentation

The six basic levels of physician segmentation are:

1. Doctors according to their age group
2. Doctors according to their specialty, such as surgeons, gynecologists, cardiologists, etc
3. General practitioners treat most patients with a particular illness, common diseases, minor ailments, etc.

4. Doctors according to the place where they practice. E.g., Urban, Rural, Government hospitals, Primary Health Centers, Private Nursing Homes, Corporate Hospitals
5. Doctors according to the type of practice. E.g. Prescribing doctors, dispensing doctors, etc.
6. Doctors according to the usage or prescribing rate. E.g., Heavy-users, light users, non-users, past-users

Patient Segmentation

The importance and significance of patient segmentation are evident from what Dr. Mickey Smith, author of Pharmaceutical Marketing, said, *it is more important to know what sort of a patient has a disease than what sort of disease a person has.*

The four basic levels of patients segmentation are:

1. Patients with similar illnesses fall under the same therapeutic group, such as diabetic patients, asthmatic patients, tuberculous patients, etc.
2. Patients can be classified depending on the stage at which the illness or disease progresses, such as, patients with acute or chronic bronchial asthma, or patients with mild, moderate, or severe hypertension.
3. Patients according to their age group such as pediatric patients, geriatric patients, etc.
4. Patients can be segmented according to gender— male and female patients

Implications for the Marketer

The needs of a physician, who is a user, and another doctor, who is a non-user, is different. The physician, who is a user (whether prescriber or dispensing), is currently satisfied with your products and their benefits. You don't have to sell the benefits and advantages of your products to him. He requires continuous reassurance that choosing your product over others has been the right decision, and is worth continuing. In other words, your communication objective is to ensure continuous usage through positive reinforcement. Whereas a physician, who is a non-user, is yet to be convinced regarding the benefits your products offer to his patients. He does not believe your product can provide the satisfaction he seeks for his patients. He needs more information with substantial evidence. He needs positive proof and outcomes from the various clinical trials conducted by eminent physicians in different hospitals of repute.

Let us now take the case of a 'past user' of your product. Your product has been coming up to his expectations in the past, but currently, he is not using your product. He needs not just information and evidence of your product's superiority over the competing ones. It would help if you investigated all the possible reasons why he stopped using your product. Is it because of competitive pressure? Or did he have any negative experience or not-so-positive experiences with the product in the recent past? Is it because of the non-availability of the product? Research in India shows that the non-availability of the products is one of the major reasons doctors give up prescribing products easily.

You can formulate your communication strategy to the 'past user' after ascertaining why he stopped using your product in the first place.

Thus, we can see that it is virtually impossible to create a single promotional communication that will satisfy the diverse needs of these three types of customers.

Similarly, based on their needs, you can formulate your communication strategies with patients suffering from different stages of similar illnesses, acute, chronic, mild, or severe.

The pharmaceutical marketer can use a segmentation strategy creatively to:

1. Identify the target group
2. Focus the promotional effort to maximize gains cost-effectively
3. Create a strong, positive product image to offset competition

Avoiding Pitfalls

While segmenting, if you maintain the essential criterion for effective segmentation, you will not likely commit the mistakes others have. Remember the following pitfalls of segmentation and always avoid them:

1. Choosing the wrong segment, which is not viable, too small, less attractive, and declining.
2. Choosing a segment that is too small and over-crowded with the competition. Such a market is fragmented rather than segmented.
3. Positioning your product as a last resort, an alternative when the leading brands fail, or as a second line of treatment. That would limit its usage rate. You can position your brand as an essential replacement to the brand leader but not as an alternative. It is not worth playing second fiddle.
4. Entering an over-crowed segment when you cannot unambiguously and perceptibly differentiate your product.

Insights are Important

The dictionary defines *insight* as penetrating mental vision or discernment. It's a faculty of seeing into inner character or underlying truth. Also, *insight* is an instance of apprehending the true nature of a thing, especially through intuitive understanding.

Now, let's look at a more practical and actionable *insight* definition. Marcus Saba and Hillary Gentile define insight in their book, Brand Plan Rx, as *the deep-seated need, fear, tension, frustration, wish, or desire that captures a not-yet obvious driver of behavior, a deep inner truth from the customer's perspective*. Thus, the insight unlocks an opportunity to inspire customer action and win in the market.

When your brand thoroughly understands its target audience by uncovering insights, it gains a significant competitive advantage. In addition, such an understanding will enable your brand to meet its unmet needs better and resonate, resulting in a better customer experience and brand loyalty. Nike's *Find Your Greatness* campaign is a classic example of how the company tapped into the powerful insight that people want to push themselves to their potential.

But how do you gain insights? Insights can come from multiple sources, such as quantitative surveys, qualitative interviews, in-home ethnographic studies, online focus groups, social listening, and conversations with patient advocacy groups (PAGs) and HCP advisory boards. However, a word of caution is in order. You cannot uncover by merely listening and conversing. In addition, you need to mine deeper to understand what people are feeling or what they believe but might not say. You need to be alert to understand what they are saying and not. As Simon Sine, the author of *Start with the Why*, says, *keep digging into the why, not the what*.

Pharmaceutical companies have always relied on physician insights mainly to promote their brands. However, while the physicians' insights are very important, it is equally, if not more important, to have a broader perspective of which pain points need to be addressed as strategic input from the start.

To gain patient insights, mapping out the patient journey is vital. However, remember that a patient journey is brand-agnostic while mapping out a patient journey. You should look for three things mainly while mapping out a patient journey:

- the level of unmet need
- the ability of your brand to address that unmet need meaningfully, and
- how it impacts your business once you deliver on that unmet need

The following table presents some examples of insights gained from patient journey mapping.

Table 1.1 Brand Insights Examples

Brand	Observation	Insight
Topamax (Topiramate)	Migraine sufferers want to reduce the frequency and severity of attacks.	It's not an attack. It's a condition.
Aciphex (Rabiprazole)	Reflux patients want symptom relief that is fast and effective.	The symptoms that no one talks about are the ones that bother reflux sufferers most.
Requip (Ropinirole)	Poor sleep plagues people as they age, and restless legs syndrome (RLS) is often the major compliant.	There Is more to *restless* than sleep.
Cialis (Tadalafil)	Has Slower onset of action, but longer duration of action (thirty-six hours).	ED (Erectile Dysfunction) is not just one person's disease; it impacts men's partners as well. Couples wanted to regain relationship by having intimacy, not only having sex.

(Source: Adapted from the Ebook, Brand Plan Rx: The Marketer's Guide to Building a Thriving Health and Wellness Brand by Markus Saba and Hillary Gentile, Bright Media)

The following three cases show how patient insights helped two big pharma firms position their brands, differentiate them from the competition, and effectively communicate to their target audience.

CASE

3

The Power of Patient Personas Extends the Brand Reach to Other Segments!

Eli Lilly and Company's segmentation and targeting of patients for launching their antidepressant Cymbalta (duloxetine) is a classic example of how to segment and target patients for marketing a prescription drug brand.

After the introduction of their highly successful antidepressant, Prozac (fluoxetine), many new SSRIs (Selective Serotonin Reuptake Inhibitors), such as Paxil (paroxetine of GlaxoSmithKline), Zoloft (Sertraline of Pfizer), and Celexa (citalopram of Forest Labs) came to market throughout the 1990s, making it a large class and highly competitive at the same time.

The brand team at Eli Lilly & Company began a massive market research program that included qualitative and quantitative surveys to gain a deep understanding of patient's needs, wants, preferences, behaviors, and characteristics. Based on this exhaustive research, the team identified seven unique, distinct, identifiable patient groups and created seven personas with their psychographic profiles representing each group. The following table presents a summary of these personas' profiles.

These patient profiles were identified, describing in detail the demographics, treatment history, current disease presentation, and other characteristics for each patient segment, quantifying the size of every segment.

Table 1.2 Patient Personas For Positioning Cymbalta

Persona	Description
Functioning Fran	Average Age. 39 Average length of depression. 5 years With anxiety symptoms. 60% With any pain symptom. 24% Top Primary Rx. Fluoxetine, Citalopram • Easy to treat, with long term remission expected • Mild severity of depression and symptoms • Younger, much less chronic and higher functioning • Very compliant
Addicted Denise	Average age 37 years Average length of depression. 7 years Top Primary Rx Fluoxetine, Bupropion With anxiety symptoms 86% With any pain symptom. 35% • Abuses drugs and alcohol • Smokes • Many co-morbidities and external stressors • Poor compliance
Complex Carl	Average age. 46 years Average length of depression. 10 years With anxiety symptoms. 95% With any pain symptoms. 68% Top Primary Rx. SSRIs, Venlafaxine • Higher number and severity of depressive symptoms • More likely to have co-morbid psychotic features, bipolar disorder, or borderline personality • Very chronic with multiple therapies • Very often considered *very difficult to treat* with lower expectations for improvement • Suspected poor compliance
Anxious Anne	Average age. 49 years Average length of depression. 7 years With anxiety symptoms. 82% With any pain symptom. 34% Top Primary RX Fluoxetine, Sertraline

Table 1.2 *Contd...*

Persona	Description
Hurting Helen	Average age 54 years Average length of depression. 9 years With anxiety symptoms 86% With any pain symptom. 100% Top Primary Rx Fluoxetine, Sertraline • Always pain, typically severe, and often fatigue or low energy symptoms • Older, longer length of suffering • More likely to be overweight and female • Somewhat difficult to treat, lower expectations on outcome, and consumes more than average healthcare resources • Disability more common
Complex Carl	Average age. 46 years Average length of depression. 10 years With anxiety symptoms. 95% With any pain symptoms. 68% Top Primary Rx. SSRIs, Venlafaxine • Higher number and severity of depressive symptoms • More likely to have co-morbid psychotic features, bipolar disorder, or borderline personality • Very chronic with multiple therapies • Very often considered *very difficult to treat* with lower expectations for improvement • Suspected poor compliance
Classic Carol	Average age. 44 years Average length of depression 7 years With anxiety symptoms. 89% With any pain symptom. 42% Top Primary Rx. Paroxetine, Citalopram • Many classic depression symptoms i.e., restlessness, appetite change, anhedonia, concentration problems, worry, guilt, irritability, nervousness, low energy, etc. • Some symptoms, but not all may be severe • Average severity overall • Fewer regimens, less length of depression suffered • Viewed as easy to treat, consuming fewer resources, with remission expected

Table 1.2 *Contd...*

Persona	Description
Non-Responding Nancy	Average age. 47 years Average length of depression. 10 years With any anxiety symptoms. 86% With any pain symptom 42% Top Primary Rx: Fluoxetine, Citalopram, Venlafaxine • Considered to be Treatment Resistant Depression (TRD) • Very chronic with multiple therapies • More severe overall and in classic depressive symptoms • Considered *Difficult to Treat* with lower expectations for improvement • Frequent combination therapy • Suspected poor compliance

The team then identified the most appropriate patient segment, *Hurting Helen*, whose unmet need ideally matched with Cymbalta's differential advantage of treating painful physical symptoms associated with Depression. Unfortunately, the Hurting Helen segment represented only eight percent of the patient population, creating doubts about the viability of a very small niche segment.

The brand team at Lilly is faced with the classic dilemma— should they select a target market for their brand that fits perfectly but is relatively very small, or do they select a target that is larger but not an ideal match with the brand's attributes?

The team debated and researched further, revealing that painful physical symptoms also show up in other patient segments. Accordingly, the team decided to focus on the *Hurting Helens* segment, which is eight percent of the market, and on patients whose main symptoms were the painful physical symptoms of Depression.

This positioning decision proved right, and the messaging resonated with the Hurting Helen segment with positive outcomes. Regarding the patients in the other segments presenting with painful physical symptoms of Depression, their physicians did not associate them with Depression. Armed with this key insight, the team developed a direct-to-customer campaign— *Depression Hurts, Cymbalta Can Help*—to help doctors recognize painful physical symptoms and associate them with Depression. In addition, it informed people of the painful physical symptoms associated with Depression and educated consumers on the link to Depression and how Cymbalta could help. The tagline, *Depression hurts, but you don't have to,* reinforces the sentiment perfectly.

As a result of the significant success that Cymbalta had with the *Hurting Helen* segment, the brand's credibility extended its reach to other segments, such as *Functioning Fran* and *Complex Carl,* with doctors putting other patients with painful physical symptoms on Cymbalta.

(Source: Adapted from the book, Brand Plan Rx: The Marketer's Guide to Building a Thriving health and Wellness Brand, by Markus Saba & Hilary GentileBrightWing Media, 2021, and Eli Lilly: Developing Cymbalta, Harvard Business School Case by Elie Ofek, Ron Laufer)

CASE

4

Topamax Has And Claims What The Patients Need And Want!

Janssen Pharmaceuticals, a subsidiary of Johnson & Johnson, a global pharma major, developed Topamax (topiramate), an anticonvulsant, and obtained US FDA approval in 1996.

Later, Janssen found that Topamax effectively prevents migraine attacks in adults and got FDA approval in 2004.

While Topamax is effective in reducing the frequency of the likelihood of migraine attacks, the patients suffering from migraine attacks did not perceive that as an unmet need worth changing their behavior. They got used to migraines as they arrived, and had prescription products to control them. In addition, they felt they knew when the migraines would happen (aura), so they preferred to continue their current regimen.

The Topamax brand team looked at the patient journey to understand their deeper feelings and needs. For example, all the migraine patients talked about the important days they would miss because of a migraine and felt that the migraine *hijacked* their life. After thoroughly analyzing the data, the brand team realized that Topamax reduced the number of migraine days. It was a *eureka* moment for the team. Fortunately, Topamax's core strength was what the patients needed. Greater control of migraine days, *not* preventing the number of attacks. The Topamax brand team could unlock an emotional driver that the brand could deliver.

While other migraine prevention treatments could also address this, no other brand has claimed this benefit and presented it compellingly, matching what the brand has with the patients' needs!

(Source: Adapted from Source: Markus Saba & Hilary Gentile, Brand Plan Rx: The Marketer's Guide to Building a Thriving health and Wellness Brand, BrightWing Media, 2021)

CASE

5

Insight-mining Helps a Third-in-Class Drug Win the Race!

In 1988, Pfizer removed the stigma around male impotence by creating a condition, Erectile Dysfunction, and launched Viagra (sildenafil) to treat it. The company aptly chose Viagra as the brand name, as Viagra suggests vitality, virility, and vigor. In addition, the name rhymes with Niagara, hinting a force and endurance. Finally, the name seems to draw inspiration from the Sanskrit word, *Vyaghra*, which means tiger.

At the launch, Pfizer positioned Viagra for erectile dysfunction in male demographics with a promise— *Go back to your former manhood*.

After five years, Rivals emerged, ready to give Viagra a fight. First was Levitra (vardenafil), developed by GlaxoSmithKline and Bayer. GlaxoSmithKline launched Levitra in the US in September 2003.

Two months later, Lilly ICOS launched Cialis (tadalafil) to treat erectile dysfunction, competing with the firmly established Viagra, with $1.8 billion in global sales, great brand equity, and outstanding customer loyalty.

The Cialis team at Lilly knew they had to position Cialis differently to steal the market share from Viagra.

The Cialis difference starts with the name itself. The root word of Cialis is *Ciel*, a French word that means *Sky* and *Heaven*.

The initial feedback from the stakeholders on the perceived clinical effects of Cialis was not encouraging. While Viagra worked fast and lasted only four hours, the slower onset of action seemed like a drawback, although it had a longer duration of action. In addition, Viagra was perceived as powerful and effective, exactly what you want to succeed in the erectile dysfunction (ED) market.

The team took a step back, studied ED (Erectile Dysfunction) more closely, examined the patient's journey, and uncovered a unique insight. They understood ED is not just one person's disease; it also impacts men's partners. They held deeper conversations with couples who said they loathed the idea of getting on with it as soon as the man was ready, as Viagra's action lasted only a few hours. During the interviews, they said *it felt like there were three of us in the bedroom: him, me, and Viagra. Once he took the pill, the clock started, and we knew we only had a few hours*.

That clue led to a deeper understanding of the partners' frustrations. What was presumed to be a disadvantage of Cialis (slower onset and longer duration of action) was a great advantage, and the short duration of Viagra (a window of opportunity that lasted only four hours) became a vulnerability. Compared to this, Cialis's thirty-six-hour duration of action is a boon to partners facing the ED problem.

The Cialis team at Eli Lilly came up with the insight that spontaneity is the key to true intimacy. Couples wanted to regain their relationship by having intimacy, not only by having sex. And for most couples, the weekend or a weekend getaway is when they truly relax and enjoy being intimately together. So, Cialis gave the couple this freedom compared to the pressure of having sex within a four-hour window after taking Viagra. That is why Cialis, in France, was colloquially referred to as *Le weekender* (the Weekender pill). Cialis reinforced this perception of intimacy and romance instead of sex only, through creative advertising.

Viagra was marketing to men and selling erections. On the contrary, Cialis was marketing to couples, intimacy, relationships, and romance. The difference is clear.

As a result of its insightful positioning that is distinctly different from the entrenched leader, Viagra, Cialis overtook Viagra as the market leader in 2013.

(Source: Adapted from Source: Markus Saba & Hilary Gentile, Brand Plan Rx: The Marketer's Guide to Building a Thriving health and Wellness Brand, BrightWing Media, 2021)

Understanding the Competition

What the great Chinese general and military strategist Sun Tzu said two thousand five hundred years ago rings true— to beat the enemy, you must understand them intimately. Once you determine who your core competitors are, you must step into their shoes and think like them to deeply understand them. Here are the key steps:

1. Firstly, define and determine who your core competitors are, what they are doing, how they are doing what they are doing and how their customers perceive them. In other words, do a competitive simulation.
2. After establishing the current state, predict, forecast, and anticipate their next moves—launches, indications, strategies, initiatives, new promotional campaigns, etc.
3. Anticipate new competitors who are not in the marketplace yet but have assets in development or pending regulatory approval.
4. Find out what other treatments the patients use, including non-medicinal interventions such as physiotherapy, exercise, over-the-counter medicines, and alternative medicines, because this is your indirect competition.

Monitoring Competition

Competitive analysis is not a one-time exercise. Therefore, you should continuously monitor the activities spanning all functional areas, and all products across geographies. Here are some key questions:

- How large and competent is their sales force?
- Do they have established relationships with KOLs (Key Opinion Leaders)?
- Which therapeutic areas are they very strong in, and will defend with all their might?
- How vested are they in the disease state? Which is their core therapeutic area, and their core business, like Novo Nordisk and diabetes, or is it only a part of their portfolio like AstraZeneca and Sanofi and Diabetes?

- Do they upgrade their technological infrastructure and manufacturing facilities constantly?
- How many of their manufacturing facilities are approved by international regulatory authorities worldwide?
- Do they have many clinical studies underway?
- What is their new product pipeline?
- Do they attend all key conferences and medical congresses?
- What is their financial status? Do they have deep pockets to put behind the brand, or are they struggling to allocate resources to other brands they have in their pipeline?
- Are they big investors in sales and marketing?
- What are their core competencies?
- Do they have a strong social media presence?
- What is their commitment to digitally transforming their organization?
- What is their organizational structure? Are they hierarchical or horizontal?
- What is their investment in R&D and technology?

Focus on two or three core competitors for analyzing deeply and monitoring continuously, not all competitors. Avoid the temptation to include every competitor in your analysis. How do you arrive at identifying your core competitors? Apart from ranking by sales and prescriptions, it is important to identify them based on customer (physician) and consumer (patient) perceptions. The key questions to ask are— If your target doctor or target patient is choosing medicine or solution, which is the main product on their mind? Which is the one that your brand would replace in their mind, and why? That's what you should consider and focus on.

Competitive Simulation

Create three cross-functional groups with persons from brand management, manufacturing, R&D, finance, MLR (medical, legal, and regulatory), and commercial to prepare brand plans for the three core competitors. Remember that you must think like your competitors and draw brand and annual marketing plans as to how they would compete against your brand. Such a simulating exercise will help you understand your competitors much deeper and anticipate their moves well in advance.

Understanding Your Brand

Whether launching new brands or managing the in-market brands, you should know your brands inside out.

In the case of new brand launches, you should go to your research and development colleagues who have been living the science, the protocols, and the trials and understand the science. The key questions are:

- How is our molecule different from competitors'?
- Does its mechanism of action yield a new treatment algorithm, or a way to approach the disease?

Once you thoroughly understand the drug's science, understand how the brand can address the patient's unmet needs and pain points. Then, for a moment, take out your industry hat, put on your customer hat, and think like an HCP, patient, and payer to understand how your new asset differs from what is currently on the market.

Review and assess your current positioning strategy for an existing brand to find whether it is still relevant to the customers' and consumers' needs and sustain its differentiation from the competition.

When assessing your brand features, advantages, and benefits, ask yourself these questions to fine-tune them.

- *Features*: What specific attributes of your brand meet a customer need the competition cannot, or has not addressed?
- *Advantage*: What functional benefit does your brand offer, and what does your brand do for the consumer and customer? What is its unique value?
- *Benefit:* What do your consumers and customers feel about the functional benefit, and what does it do to them?

These insights into your target customers can help you determine a precise positioning for your brand. The following table presents a few examples of these concepts.

Table 1.3 Features, Advantages, and Benefits: Some Examples

Brand / Company	Features	Advantages	Benefits
Topamax (Topiramate, Janssen)	Reduces frequency of migraine attacks	Fewer days with migraines	Prevents migraines from hijacking your life
Cialis (Tadalafil, Lilly ICOS)	Has thirty-six hour efficacy	Grants longer time frame in which to initiate sex	Restores intimacy— when the moment is right
Nexium (Esomeprazole, AstraZeneca)	Utilizes superior healing data	Not only treats reflux symptoms but heals the damage	Fixes the underlying problem

Source: Markus Saba & Hilary Gentile, Brand Plan Rx: The Marketer's Guide to Building a Thriving health and Wellness Brand, BrightWing Media, 2021)

It's not enough to create differentiation while positioning. You must communicate the *difference* effectively.

What the late Professor Theodore Levitt said about features and benefits long ago rings true. He said people don't buy your features and attributes; they buy the benefits they offer. He said, for example, when a customer is purchasing your two-inch drilling machine, he is not buying the machine; he is buying a two-inch hole!

Typology of Benefits

A product's benefits are of three types— Functional, Rational, and Emotional.

1. *Functional Benefits* are based on the product's attributes and features. These are differentiated aspects of the products supported by data and evidence, such as efficacy, safety, dosing, mechanism of action (MOA), and side effects.
2. *Rational benefits* are the consequences of the attributes to the stakeholders, such as patients, doctors, and payers. Rational benefits explain why functional benefits matter to customers

and consumers. For example, functional benefits like better efficacy, fewer side effects, and more convenient dosing could mean improved adherence and compliance, leading to better patient outcomes. Thus, rational benefits help the brand differentiate itself from the competition and become more meaningful to customers and consumers.

3. Though intangible, *Emotional benefits* result from rational benefits and make customers think and feel about the brand. Emotional benefits are not based on hard data or evidence. They come from your insights research that includes talking to customers and listening to them intently about what they are saying and not saying. Examples of emotional benefits include how Eli Lilly built their Cialis brand and Merck their Fosamax brand.

Research has shown that emotional benefits are more important in improving brand conversions and loyalty than rational benefits, even for prescription drug brands. Although physicians rely heavily on scientific data, they are still human beings full of emotions. Therefore, those with a positive emotional association with your brand tend to prescribe it more and are much more brand loyal.

Therefore, communicating the differentiation's tangible, intangible, and emotional benefits is crucial in establishing your brand's position in the customer's mind. The Key questions are:

- Have you identified your brand's tangible, intangible, and emotional benefits?
- What are the key differentiators of your brand from what the competition offers? Is it relevant to customers' functional and emotional needs? Do customers value them enough to choose your brand over competitors'?
- Can you substantiate your differentiation? Do you have compelling evidence and scientific data to support this?

Here's a case that shows how AstraZeneca communicated its brand differentiation single-mindedly.

CASE

6

Winning with Communication as the Key Differentiator!

AstraZeneca launched its statin brand, Crestor (rosuvastatin), in the US in 2003. Till the launch of Crestor, the main focus of most statins has been on their ability to lower total cholesterol. However, AstraZeneca differentiated its message from the rest of the statins from the beginning of Crestor's launch. The company differentiated between *good* cholesterol (HDL) and *bad* cholesterol (LDL), focusing its messaging on Crestor's ability to increase good cholesterol while lowering bad cholesterol (LDL). The superiority of Crestor's power to reduce LDL is backed by evidence. For example, Crestor reduced LDL by 55 percent, while Lipitor (Atorvastatin) reduced it by 43 percent and Zocor (simvastatin) by 38 percent.

Having found its secret sauce, which is Crestor's power to reduce bad cholesterol (LDL), AstraZeneca sharpened its message focus with a single-minded proposition of *fighting bad cholesterol*. As a result, the company, being the first to market with this data with clear and distinct arrows pointing down and stating that Crestor lowers bad cholesterol and by how much, became very successful.

(Source: Adapted from the book, Brand Plan Rx: The Marketer's Guide to Building a Thriving health and Wellness Brand, by Markus Saba & Hilary GentileBrightWing Media, 2021)

Competitive SWOT Analysis

SWOT analysis seems to be ubiquitous in today's business world, with every brand and annual marketing plan containing a SWOT analysis. For example, when you type SWOT in Google, over 22 million results pop up, says Beata Borucka in her book, *SWOT & So What: Make Sense of Your Plans.*

The SWOT analysis is a look at your brand's Strengths (S), Weaknesses (W), Opportunities (O), and threats (T).

Most SWOT analyses are not more than an arbitrary list of strengths, weaknesses, threats, and opportunities and therefore are not actionable.

To gain actionable insights, you must match a Strength to a market or consumer opportunity. You must also evaluate Weaknesses and threats by listing out weaknesses identified by your marketing team and then comparing them with the list of threats the company faces or may face from competing products or the market itself. When you do this, your Weaknesses and Strengths will tell you what actions you need to take to prevent getting attacked from unexpected positions.

Making SWOT Actionable

Beata Borucka, a marketing strategist and SWOT analysis expert, suggested a revolutionary way of analyzing SWOT to make it actionable in her book, *SWOT, So What*:

While SWOT analysis contains many details, there is no clear conclusion, call to action, or actionable plan. To make your SWOT analysis actionable, consider the following steps.

- In the classic SWOT grid, the left-hand column (Strengths and Opportunities) shows how you can grow your brand, and the right-hand column (Weaknesses and Threats) points to the challenges you face in growing your brand.
- Do not look for a ready or quick SWOT analysis. Do not fill the Opportunities area in the grid with feel-good and obvious ideas.

Instead, review the data, your knowledge, your experiences, and your feelings to arrive at a meaningful, actionable SWOT analysis.

- The first step to SWOT analysis is to look at the information you have acquired and to split them into internal data (Strengths and Weaknesses) and external data (Threats and Opportunities). In other words, sort these internal data into our strengths and weaknesses and market information on Opportunities and Threats. In Opportunities, there are ideas for actions and options for solutions for the company's problems and perceived Threats.
- In Opportunities, most SWOT analyses list ambitious ideas or obvious solutions like desired answers to threats. In Threats, there are usually hysterical comments about cost containment, stringent government price regulations, the inflow of cheap generics, etc.
- Instead, we need to analyze these objectively and specifically by sorting the internal data under the marketing-mix elements (4Ps—Product, Promotion, Place, and Price) into strengths and weaknesses to find actionable answers and solutions. Likewise, you need to sort the data from the customers' and market's perspective into Opportunities and Threats. Analyzing our Strengths and Weaknesses from a 4P perspective introduces order and logic in thinking and discussions.
- The key question to ask is —What are our strengths? What distinguishes us, is essential, and allows us to grow?
- While filling the SWOT grid, your answers to Who and What is your company and brand will clarify your Strengths, Weaknesses, Opportunities, and Threats. For example, if the answers to the question of Who and What is your company and brand, that is undoubtedly a Strength or Weakness. If your answer to the question of Who and What is the market or customer, that is the Opportunities and Threats area.

It would be best if we do a SWOT analysis for our major competing brands to win in today's hyper-competitive market place.

7 Ps and 7 Cs

The marketing mix elements help us reflect on essential business areas in a systematic, orderly manner from the company's internal perspective. So let's start with the first P, the Product.

Do we have a distinguishing feature with the core product? How differentiated is it? With the opportunities for differentiating the core product increasingly diminishing, can we look into the other marketing mix elements, such as promotion, packaging, price, etc., to differentiate our product?

So far, we have organized our data from the **"P"** perspective (Producer or manufacturer's point of view) to look at our market opportunities. As a second step, let's examine the marketing environment to define our market opportunities and identify risks or threats. You can understand the marketing environment only when you analyze it from the customers' perspective. Philip Kotler, the venerated marketing guru, suggests the view of the potential or customer, that is, external factors. The customer lens looks like this:

- The *Product* turns into *Customer Value* for our market's stakeholders.
- *Price* turns into *Cost* that buyer is ready to pay for their value or need.
- The *Place* turns into *Convenience*, which means the convenience of purchase.
- *Promotion* turns into *Communication* or dialogue with the market.
- *People* turn into *Confidence* creating our people in touch with the market.
- *Processes* turn into the *Comfort* of buying our goods.
- *Physical Evidence* turns into *Credibility* we must build in our customers' minds.

The first **"C"** in external factors, an analogy to the product in the internal analysis, concerns the customer's expectations for products in each category. It is defined as *Customer Value*, which is the value the customer is looking for in a product or service.

Maybe there are some Customer Values your product can meet today or later after modifying it appropriately to suit the customers' wants and unmet needs. The place for such observations is in the Opportunities field in your SWOT analysis grid.

It is important to remember that when defining Opportunities and Threats, we should also look at them from the customer's perspective by walking in her shoes.

In this SWOT analysis, Strengths and Weaknesses are arranged through the 4 Ps (Product, Place, Promotion, and Price), and opportunities and Threats through the 4 Cs (Customer Value, Convenience, Communication, and Cost) to make to actionable.

SWOT Matrix: A New Lens

SWOT analysis helps us plan actions and shows us the logic and legitimacy of our choices. It also plays an important role in obtaining the consent of the decision-makers for the proposed activities and budget approvals. However, it would be best if you had a new lens to see these and create a SWOT matrix by reversing the table layout and assigning internal sales analysis records to an external analysis. Only such an exercise will enable findings and suggestions to become actionable. The following table presents an overview of the SWOT Matrix through a new lens.

Table 1.4 SWOT Analysis Through A New Lens

Strengths	Weaknesses
How to Grow? Growth Strategy	What to Improve Development Strategy
How to defend oneself? Defense Strategy	How not to get killed? Survival Strategy

(Source: Adapted from the book, SWOT So What by Beata Borucka, EXertus Group, 2018)

SWOT Analysis: Points to Ponder

Finally, four points to ponder when you do a SWOT analysis to get the most out of it.

1. Identify which of our strengths will allow us to defend ourselves against threats and what is worth improving to take advantage of existing opportunities.
2. We must prepare well for the threats related to our weaknesses because if we do not address them, the consequences can be critical even to our functioning.
3. A clear, unambiguous product positioning for our brand is crucial for our development strategy as it sets the pace for the rest of the activities, starting from communication.
4. Developing insights into what can help us look at the opportunities in the market that we can use and what will let us defend ourselves.
5. Sometimes, it is more important to decide what we will stop doing than what we will do. Because as Peter Drucker, the father of modern management, said: *one of the worst decisions in business is doing the wrong things right*.

Differential Advantage

Uniqueness or perceived uniqueness is a product's only protection against commodity status, which means the product is being bought solely on price criterion.

In the case of prescription drug brands, patents further strengthen the uniqueness at least as long as the patent lasts. Therefore, creating a perceptible differential advantage is essential to position your brand. If you do not recognize and realize the importance of positioning and position your products, it can lead to:

- your new products failing in the market without generating adequate sales and profits, or
- the new products may succeed but at the expense of other products (illusion of success and cannibalization)

Therefore, the understanding of differentiation and positioning is crucial for success in marketing your products successfully. David Aaker emphasized the indispensable role of positioning in marketing when he said: *Product positioning is so central and critical that it should be considered at the mission statement level as it represents the essence of business*.

3 Fundamental Criteria

Your product offering should satisfy three fundamental criteria to create a differential advantage.

- It differentiates the product from all others, creating a perception of uniqueness. Also, the target audience must perceive the uniqueness as important and relevant to them.
- It is important, or can be made to seem important to the target audience.
- It is sustainable over time against the competition. Investing in a differential advantage that competitors can easily imitate and copy is not useful. Because of the distinguishing features created, the differential advantage will then simply evaporate. So, the sustainability of your differential advantage is crucial.

Each of these three criteria described above is vital in establishing a viable, sustainable positioning for the product.

Therefore, The primary task of marketers is to create a differential advantage. The secondary task is to defend it with all their might. There are two basic approaches to achieving this. One is to increase the importance of the product features or attributes and their benefits, which are perceived as unique. Alternatively, one can reduce the importance of the product features or attributes and the benefits of competitors' products, which are perceived as unique. Here are two cases highlighting these two approaches.

CASE

7

The Fabulous Success Story of American Remedies in the Systemic Anti-Fungal Market!

American Remedies, one of the fastest-growing companies in the Indian pharmaceutical industry, spotted an opportunity in the early 1990s (Dr. Reddy's Laboratories later acquired the company) in the systemic anti-fungal market. Griseofulvin was the most widely prescribed anti-fungal for systemic use (77 percent of the market in 1992). However, only two companies - IDPL and Glaxo with its two brands (Grisovin FP and Dermonorm)— had accounted for over two-thirds of the total anti-fungal market. As a small company, American Remedies could not have thought of succeeding with another brand of griseofulvin in the systemic anti-fungal market. So it had to do something different— a perceivable differential advantage over the other brands of griseofulvin, and brands of emerging new anti-fungal molecules like ketoconazole, etc.

After a thorough inquiry into the perceptions and the needs of the target consumers and users, the company identified a vacant, unoccupied slot in the perceptual space of the target consumers— the convenience of dosage. The recommended dosage for all griseofulvin brands was one tablet four times a day. When you consider the patients' pain point was the low levels of gastric tolerance associated with griseofulvin coupled with a Four-times-daily dosage regimen, a vacant slot suddenly becomes obvious, and what other companies were oblivious to, became obvious to American Remedies.

The company found out that it could offer a once-a-day griseofulvin brand by reducing the particle size further, down to about 400 microns. The company introduced Gris OD (griseofulvin once daily) and communicated this differential advantage forcefully and persuasively. As a result, the convenient dosage regime became far more important to the prescribing physicians. This differential advantage of the once-a-day brand of the well-established griseofulvin molecule paved the way for the dramatic success of Gris OD. The brand achieved a leadership position in the systemic anti-fungal market soon enough.

A seemingly simple, even obvious positioning slot can result in fabulous success when exploited well!

CASE

8

Undermining Others' Differential Advantage?

Zantac's pre-emptive strike against Losec (now Prilosec) offers an excellent example of undermining the differential advantage created by potential competitors. Zantac (ranitidine) of Glaxo (GSK now) had achieved the distinction of being the world's largest prescription drug brand (sales US $2.7 billion in 1991-92). Losec (omeprazole), an original research product of Astra, belongs to a different class of drugs (proton pump inhibitor) even though it is in the same therapeutic category of anti-ulcerants. Losec offers a distinct advantage in faster ulcer healing and low (if not absent) relapse rates. Glaxo sensing this, decided to undermine the differential advantage and launched a pre-emptive strike against Losec internationally, creating a dissonance among the prescribers. It succeeded in making Losec a reserve drug for some time as a second-line treatment.

Meanwhile, Glaxo pursued a market development strategy by expanding the usage of Zantac in non-ulcer dyspepsia, gastritis, etc. Glaxo could do this primarily from its preeminent position. It had built up a lot of credibility. Astra (AstraZeneca now) had also built up a lot of substantial clinical evidence and got in Prilosec cleared as a first-line drug in gastric ulcers.

Glaxo surely had bought time by undermining the differential advantage created by Astra and defended its leadership position for Zantac in the anti-ulcer wars!

Unfortunately, although pharmaceutical research differentiates their products with intrinsic qualities like better safety profile, increased efficacy, and longer duration of action, the differential advantage is short-lived. This is because patents can only protect the differential advantage until the patents last, ten to twelve years from launch or twenty years from the filing date. So, pharma marketers would do better by differentiating their product (in addition to intrinsic differentiation) in relatively underexploited attributes such as brand name, color, form, size or shape, packaging, taste, consistency, etc, to create a unique perception. For example, Migraleve, a migraine product in the UK, became popular for reasons other than therapeutic effects. Its success is because Migraleve has developed its tablet in appealing pink color and an attractive package differentiating it from the rest.

In other industries, many examples of uniqueness are not based on product features and benefits. Consider these, for example:

- IBM's uniqueness is its size
- HeinekenBeer's advertising image is unique, especially in the US and UK. Coca-Cola's uniqueness worldwide is its distribution system and American origins.

However, these non-product uniqueness opportunities are not yet fully exploited in the pharmaceutical industry. While government regulation is a limiting factor on claims and positioning in the prescription drug industry, there will still be opportunities for various other positioning strategies.

The following cases show companies using non-product uniqueness to differentiate their brands achieved success.

CASE

9

The Silent Salesman Adds Value!

An example of product augmentation by packaging is Lederle's (Pfizer now) Prenatal capsules in the 1960s in India. Prenatal capsules are hematinic capsules specially meant for pregnant women, as the name suggests. The name tells it all. They brought about an innovative and voluntary improvement in the packaging. They introduced a very attractive and innovative pack of 120 capsules for their Prenatal capsules in the shape of a feeding bottle, which is reusable. It also ensured that the consumer bought 120 capsules at a time. The product did very well with this packaging innovation. This would have probably taken the brand further up, even to a leadership position. But, the company took the pressure off this product, and the brand slipped from its rank and market share. Prenatal was a brand to reckon with in its heydays. The silent salesman did add value!

CASE

10

Innovation Makes All the Difference!

Another example of product augmentation is Fefol, the pregnancy hematinic from SmithKline French, known as Eskay Labs in India (GlaxoSmithKline now). Fefol was no more than a hematinic formulation containing 150 mg of ferrous sulfate and 0.5 mg of folic acid. Nothing was exciting about the formulation. There were many hematinic formulations containing these two ingredients in even higher quantities. But the product augmentation was achieved in Fefol by its superior formulation, which is the forerunner of new drug delivery systems sweeping the pharmaceutical market today. Even the presentation of the product was distinctly different. It was a different kind of capsule called a *Spansule*, which contained the active ingredients in the form of tiny pellets—hundreds of them inside each transparent capsule. These pellets are coated especially to ensure timed disintegration. Apart from its technical benefits, the product is a beautiful see-through capsule with hundreds of multi-colored time-release pellets. The benefit: freedom from side effects associated with oral iron therapy. They have dramatically, effectively, and persuasively communicated this benefit package to doctors in the country. In addition, they introduced a new brand, Fesovit (iron with multivitamins), in the same *spansule* form of capsules. They promoted these brands vigorously and achieved a leadership position with a market share (combined for both Fefol and Fesovit) of 15 percent in 1999.

CASE

11

Antacid Market: Emergence of A new Leader!

Gelusil of Warner Hindusthan (now Pfizer) had been enjoying brand leadership in the Rs. 78-crore large (1992) antacid, antiflatulent market. It has been a brand leader since its launch in 1973.

Its served market had been considerably large with other prominent brands like Aludrox, Divol, Digene, etc. However, although introduced in 1968, it was only during the 1970s that Digene created a perceptible product differentiation by adding an antiflatulent (Methylpolysiloxane) and pushed the product aggressively into the competitors' territory. As a result, its volume grew, and market share moved significantly, making Digene the undisputed brand leader in 1992 with a 20 percent share of the antacid-antiflatulent market.

CASE

12

The Antacid that Neutralized Even the Competition!

A medium-sized, rapidly growing pharmaceutical company had introduced an antacid brand, 'x,' in the Rs. 44-crore large antacid, antiflatulent (actual) market. However, when you add the anti-peptic-ulcerants to this, the (potential) market becomes larger by another Rs. 31 crores (1988).

The company was well aware that the potential market (antacids, anti-flatulents, and anti-peptic ulcerants) was in its growth phase, and more than hundred brands were already fighting for their survival and growth. Therefore, introducing yet another antacid at this stage was no easy task. However, the company was determined to enter this large market as part of its product diversification strategy and to make the most of it.

The company had meticulously planned a new product with a perceptible differentiation — a new ingredient, different flavor, new additional benefits, and impactful communication package coupled with attractive sampling to induce trial and specialized training to the field force — in short, the whole works.

Besides, the company's marketing team had a stormy brainstorming session to plot the PLC (Product Life Cycle) for their product, and preempt competitors' likely moves (the top five competitors accounted for over 90 percent of the actual market) and new entrants. The launch had been a success by all standards. In less than one year, the product picked up a 2.4 percent market share, which no other antacid introduced during the preceding five years had achieved. However, the product had not made any dent in the top five brands. Being alert, ever-vigilant competitors, they responded quickly, stepped up their promotional inputs, and mounted an offensive on this fledgling brand.

Since the company had preempted and anticipated the signature moves of competitors, it did not catch itself off-guard. The company was well prepared to meet the competitive challenge. The company had plotted the PLC and the strategic action for their brand 'x.' The company's analysis was somewhat like the one presented in Table 1.5.

Table 1.5 PLC and Planning for a New Antacid Brand

1. **Introduction:** Brand 'x' should be different from all other antacids available in the market and should be perceived as such by our prospective customers. The differentiation should be created in the:
   A. Composition
   B. Shape
   C. Color
   D. Flavor
   E. Pack
   F. Promotion at the doctor level as well as at the chemist level
   G. Price-skimming strategy, though the pharmaceutical industry is subjected to the government predetermines rigorous price controls and mark-ups. Since the active ingredient in brand 'x' was not listed in any controlled categories at the time some flexibility in pricing exists.
   H. Launch itself
2. **Likely Responses of Competition:** The pharmaceutical market in India is virtually a me-too market. The possibility of new competitors joining the fray once the product is accepted is certain. The primary competitors, who are currently taking their respective market shares for granted but for a few skirmishes around the borders of their served markets, face no threats. The shares of the market leaders were more or less frozen. The success of brand 'x' might shake them out of their complacency. That would mean waking up the sleeping giants. With their resources, they can launch a major offensive. Brand 'x,' therefore, must initiate product development and product diversification strategies before the introduction so that it need not be caught napping during the crucial growth phase.
3. **Product Development:** The company and the brand 'x' better be right the first time. Since the company is fighting the international giants in the market and the target customers are educated and enlightened, qualitative differentiation (in

addition to aesthetics) is, of course, a must. Not only that, to counter the competitors' moves effectively during the growth phase, but also product development efforts should be concentrated in significant areas such as:

- Acid neutralizing capacity
- Taste. Since antacids are chewable, the flavor becomes a considerable factor.

Initiating the necessary changes to improve the product before the introduction is critical.

4. **Product Diversification:** To develop new flavors since the competitors might try to introduce different flavors. The company should be prepared to launch more brand 'x' flavors during the maturity phase (essential to maintain novelty and sustain the interest of the early majority) or earlier if the competitors' moves warrant it.

   To look for new segments and enter with necessary product modifications (like a combination of local anesthetic, the small but attractive segment) to prolong, extend and indeed avert the decline phase. The company differentiated their brand in multiple ways resulting in a successful launch.

While these may sound or look like oversimplified statements, that is what exactly happened. Moreover, the competitors' responses were indeed predictable in retrospect, for they had acted as anticipated by the company even before the introduction of its brand 'x.'

Though brand 'x' was yet to achieve the preeminent position it had set out to (the brand, as well as the market, were still in the growth phase in the early 1990s), in the final analysis, brand 'x' seemed to be successful not only in neutralizing the acid but even the competitors' offensive!

Points of Parity and Points of Differentiation

Usually, consumers evaluate brands in a particular category and narrow their choices to about three to four brands based on their screening criteria, such as previous exposure, brand awareness, price, and more, before making a final purchase decision. Peter Wright and Fredric Barbour used the term— consideration set, first in 1977. Therefore, unless your brand is among the two or three brands in the consideration set of the consumer's mind, it has no chance of succeeding in the marketplace.

Points of Parity (POP) are prerequisites to enter into the consideration set of customer when the customer is choosing which brand to purchase, while Points of Difference (POD) are the motivating factors helping him to choose a particular brand.

Consider whether your brand lacks a point of parity on key dimensions. The most compelling point of difference will not win unless parity is achieved. Like Woody Allen famously said, *80 percent of success is just showing up*. Without points of parity, you will not be showing up. It will not be seen as a relevant, preferred brand—and it will not be considered.

When analyzing the competition, you should consider Points of Parity (POP) and Points of Difference (POD). Points of parity to associate the brand with the category for easy identification by the customer and points of difference to communicate the brand's superiority. While SWOT (Strengths, Weaknesses, Opportunities, and Threats) analysis is useful in developing a brand strategy, POP and POD analysis helps arrive at a meaningful proposition demonstrating customer value. In his book *Strategic Brand Management*, Kevin Lane Keller suggests that every brand must have specific points of parity (POPs) dictated by the product category. For example, toothpaste must have good foam, an acceptable taste, and the ability to clean teeth effectively. While these are not compelling reasons for the customer to purchase, they are hygiene factors whose absence will adversely affect the purchase by customers.

Today's customers have a set of up to three or four brands for purchase consideration in their minds in a given category. A brand must have a parity perception to get into that consideration set. Once a brand is among the three or four brands in the customer's consideration set, then the points of differentiation come into play to make the final purchase decision. The stronger and more compelling the point of difference, the greater the probability of purchasing that brand. PODs motivate the customer to choose a particular brand over others. Therefore, marketers should identify PODs that are present or create them in their brand so the customer chooses them.

According to Kevin Lane Keller, the main elements of PODs (Points of Difference) are— Relevance, Desirability, Distinctiveness, Believability, Feasibility, Communicability, and Sustainability. The key questions to ask when assessing your brand's points of difference are:

- Is the POD distinctive, superior, and desirable from the customer's perspective? How relevant is the POD as a solution to the customer's pain point? For example, you promote a non-steroidal anti-inflammatory drug for its long-lasting action. When customers are looking for rapid pain relief, they may perceive it as slow to act because they may think if it is long-lasting, it must be slow-acting.
- How distinctive is the POD?
- How believable is the POD? Is the evidence compelling? Credible? Do we have adequate scientific evidence to substantiate our brand's point of difference?
- Can we deliver what we promise? Is our POD feasible? For example, it is widely acknowledged that NSAID brands cause gastric irritation, and that's why antiulcerants are mostly co-prescribed with almost all NSAID brands. So, while an NSAID without gastric irritation will be distinctly different and most desirable, is it feasible to deliver on that? Can we formulate an NSAID that does not cause gastric irritation?

- Can we communicate our brand's POD effectively, substantiating with clinical studies? For example, it isn't easy to communicate intangible benefits in therapeutic categories with no biological markers to see the difference. Presenting and publishing the patient's or caregiver's feedback on treatment is how you can communicate your POD in such cases.
- How sustainable is our point of difference? There are two aspects to sustainability. One is creating a point of difference that is difficult to imitate and copy by competitors. The other is holding on to that POD for a longer period. Usually, pharmaceutical companies start brand-related services with enthusiasm but fail to sustain them for a longer period. You should not select a POD unless you can sustain it.

The following table will be useful in identifying the points of difference (POD) between the prescription drug brands. The POD list suggested is only indicative and illustrative and not exhaustive. You can add more relevant points of differentiation based on your brand, category, and competition.

Table 1.6 Analyzing *Points of Difference* to Develop Superior Products

Our Brand	Competitor A	Competitor B	Competitor C	Difference	Relevance (of the Difference) to the Patient
Composition					
Mechanism of Action					
Efficacy					
Safety					
Adverse Reactions					
Dosage form: If it is oral, • Size of the tablet / scored or un-scored • Is it a swallow tablet or mouth dissolving • Is it a sustained-released dosage form • In case of capsule, Size of the capsule and type— hard or soft, If it is liquid form, • Syrup or Suspension • Sugar-free or not • Palatable or not					

Table 1.6 *Contd...*

Our Brand	Competitor A	Competitor B	Competitor C	Difference	Relevance (of the Difference) to the Patient
Which flavor? If it is a parenteral, • Intramuscular, or intravenous • Pain free or not If it is a topical preparation, • Ointment or solution • In case of ointment is it cream based or greasy **Manufacturing:** Is there a unique manufacturing process for this brand? Dose **Packaging:** Is it unique? Does it add any value to the brand? Duration of treatment Cost of treatment What is the Brand's Positioning?Tagline?Promotional theme? Points of Difference, and their relevance to the patient					

Table 1.6 *Contd...*

Our Brand	Competitor A	Competitor B	Competitor C	Difference	Relevance (of the Difference) to the Patient
Clinical evidence to support your points of difference How important is the brand to the company? What are the stakes? How strong or dominant is the company in this therapeutic segment? Number of HCPs targeted for the Brand's promotion **Reach**: How many HCPs are we targeting for this Brand?**Frequency**: What is the call frequency for this brand promotion?**Specialty Focus:** Which specialities are we targeting for this brand? **Marketing Mix: Number of Physicians Covered with:** • Detailing , Physical, E-Detailing • Product Symposia or Seminars—online and offline					

Table 1.6 *Contd...*

Our Brand	Competitor A	Competitor B	Competitor C	Difference	Relevance (of the Difference) to the Patient
• Any Service-around-the-pill or Beyond-the-pill activities to improve patient adherence, if relevant • Samples • Any other activity such as Disease Awareness Campaigns SWOT Analysis of the Brand Strengths: Weaknesses: Opportunities: Threats: SWOT Analysis of the Company Strengths: Weaknesses: Opportunities: Threats: **Online Presence of the Brand.** • Does the brand have a website? If so:					

Table 1.6 *Contd...*

Our Brand	Competitor A	Competitor B	Competitor C	Difference	Relevance (of the Difference) to the Patient
• No of page views • Average time on page • Average session duration • Pages per session • Bounce rate • New visitor sessions • Repeat visitors How Social is the Brand? What are the social media channels on which the brand is present? What are the metrics? • LIkes • Comments • Shares					

Types of Positioning

Pharmaceutical companies have positioned their brands mainly relying on technical aspects of the products. As long as pharma was able to develop breakthrough drugs through their research and development activity, creating a significant differential advantage, this approach has been effective. However, pharmaceutical companies recently started focusing on incremental developments over the existing molecules and patentable research for various reasons. As a result, they are unable to create a significant differential advantage. Therefore, finding alternative sources of creating differential advantages to position their brands became a necessity. For example, a breakthrough new product to cure cancer will most likely have a differential advantage. At the same time, the twenty-first anti-rheumatic drug, from a technical point of view, is not a breakthrough but a challenge to marketers. In his book, *Competitive Strategy in Pharmaceutical Marketing*, Marcel Corstenjs suggests many types of positioning for prescription drug brands.

Positioning Based On A Specific Attribute

Most pharmaceutical companies focus their positioning of prescription drug brands on specific attributes of their products, such as potency (efficacy), favorable side effect profile, and tolerance to differentiate them. For example, American Home Products (Pfizer, now) positioned its Ultradol (combination of tramadol and paracetamol) as a therapy for arthritis with lower gastrointestinal side effects and a convenient dosage regimen.

Positioning for Use, or Application

One of the popular positioning approaches is *once-daily* positioning. Many pharmaceutical companies use it as a differentiator, as convenience of dosage is an important benefit that improves adherence. Consider these examples.

- Pfizer positioned its Feldene (piroxicam) as the first once-a-day non-steroidal anti-inflammatory drug for arthritis.

- ICI's (AstraZeneca, now) Tenormin (atenolol) entered the US market as the fourth beta-blocker. However, Tenormin had two differential advantages— cardioselectivity and once-daily dosage convenience. Therefore, the company positioned Tenormin as a once-daily beta-blocker with cardioselectivity.

In addition, pharma companies also position their drugs as first-line, second-line, or third-line therapies. They can also use a positioning strategy classifying them across a broad range of galenical forms. A notable example is Voltaren, introduced as an acute anti-inflammatory in 25 mg, and 50 mg tablets, followed by an injectable form. Later Ciba-Geigy (Novartis, now) introduced Voltaren as a suppository for nighttime relief and once-daily tablets for chronic anti-inflammatory treatment. Later the company introduced Voltaren Gel, a topical preparation for localized pain.

Positioning for the End User (Type of Patient)

There are many positioning opportunities for pharma marketers, and patient, or user-based positioning is important. You can position your prescription drug brand in many ways, such as minor or major degrees of disease, acute or chronic sufferers, adults or children, old or young, or by attitudes to treat, or ethnic groups. However, avoiding the temptation to aim for all possible cases is important. Instead, focusing on the most appropriate position can help establish your brand in the prescribers' minds. Once you get a firm foothold on one position, you can expand later. Alternatively, you can also aim at a broad spectrum of applications like Glaxo (GlaxoSmithKline, now) did when it launched Zantac (ranitidine), the second H2 antagonist. Instead of attacking SmithKline Beecham's Tagamet (cimetidine), the first H2 antagonist head-on, Glaxo defined a broader target market.

Marketing to a broader segment requires more customers and, consequently, a larger field force. For example, Glaxo entered into a co-marketing alliance with Roche in the US and accessed a larger field force to promote Zantac.

Two more examples of pharmaceutical companies using end-user segmentation are:

- Bristol-Myers Squibb focused only on severe hypertensive cases for their first-in-class ACE inhibitor, Capoten (captopril).
- On the other hand, Merck Sharp and Dohme (MSD) targeted less severe cases of hypertension, a broader market segment for their ACE inhibitor Vasotec (enalapril) with a low dose composition, and took advantage of its larger field forces that enabled greater coverage.

Positioning by Competition

You can also position your brand by using competition as a reference point. It allows you to piggyback on the good image of a competitor's product, and yet differentiate your brand by adding a differential advantage. For example, Ciba-Geigy (Novartis, now) used this approach when it launched its non-steroidal anti-inflammatory drug, Rengasil (pirprofen), in France, positioning it as a more potent product in the same market where they had another product, Voltaren (diclofenac), a non-steroidal anti-inflammatory drug. Later, the company realized that the differentiation between the two brands in the market was inadequate and not as distinct as it should be to avoid cannibalization. So, the company repositioned Rengasil with an emphasis on its analgesic properties and differentiated it from Voltaren, the anti-inflammatory brand.

Positioning by Product Class

Positioning by product class, particularly when they are first-in-class, is a standard practice in pharmaceutical marketing. ICI's (AstraZeneca, now) Inderal (propranolol, the first beta-blocker), SmithKline Beecham's (GlaxoSmithKline, now), Tagamet (cimetidine, the first H2 antagonist) and Bristol-Myers Squibb's Capoten (Captopril, the first ACE inhibitor) are some notable examples for first-in-class drugs that became blockbusters.

Usually, the first-in-class brand will have a differential advantage and can be positioned as a better option than competitors' products. If you combine it with marketing excellence, the brand will become a blockbuster like Prozac (Fluoxetine, the first SSRI agent) from Eli Lilly.

But how to position a fifth-in-class drug?

The following two cases show how Prozac, a first-in-class drug, and Lipitor, a fifth-in-class drug, were successfully marketed.

CASE

13

Prozac: A Classic Example of Marketing Excellence!

In 1999, Fortune magazine added Prozac to its Products of the Century list, putting it in the company of Penicillin, Band-Aid, Radio, Television, and the World Wide Web. In response to this, Garry Tollefson, then president of neuroscience products of Eli Lilly, which discovered and developed Prozac, commented: *The recognition by Fortune underscores the critical role that Prozac has played in elevating the awareness of major depression as a disorder of the brain, the importance of seeking medical evaluation and the existence of safe and effective treatment.*

Eli Lilly introduced Prozac (Fluoxetine) to treat depression in the Un ted States in 1987. Prozac had crossed the $1 billion mark in sales, and achieved blockbuster status in 1992. Prozac had achieved more than sales and prescriptions. By 1994, Prozac's name recognition had attained Kleenex's familiarity and spring water's social status, according to an oft-quoted Newsweek piece. There is more. Twenty-five years after Prozac was introduced, the name entered the cultural lexicon and helped define how people think of mental illness. How did Prozac achieve all this?

What is behind the spectacular success of Prozac? It is Lilly's strategic marketing excellence. That is evident right from the brand name it gave to its first-in-class selective serotonin reuptake inhibitor (SSRI), Fluoxetine, Prozac— a name that is created by the internationally renowned branding firm Interbrand. A name that aimed to distance the drug from everything typically associated with antidepressants— strong chemical side effects, etc. Eli Lilly hired Interbrand to find a zesty, communicable name that cuts through the clutter for the blandly titled chemical compound - Fluoxetine hydrochloride. Finally, the company chose Prozac because *Pro* connoted positivity and professionalism, and *Zac* action.

The marketing success of Prozac was so spectacular that its marketing strategy became the standard operating procedure for subsequent psychiatric drug campaigns. Here are some of the key action steps that the company took to promote Prozac:

1. A few months before the launch of Prozac, Ken Cohen, a marketing manager at Eli Lilly, convened a series of educational meetings involving about 150 of the company's senior executives, and leading psychiatrists. This marketing move of grooming key opinion leaders (KOLs) as prominent spokespersons when a company launches a new drug to bolster its acceptability within the larger medical community has become standard practice in the pharmaceutical industry.
2. Lilly hired teams of medical representatives and meticulously prepared them to familiarize doctors with the therapeutic benefits of Prozac. The company knew if representatives were to be persuasive in changing physicians' prescribing habits, the reps would have to be more than just informed— they should have a genuine belief and one-hundred percent conviction in their product.
3. Personal relations with physicians are key to success, and the reps must develop a rapport with physicians.
4. Prozac was considered a clean drug, targeting serotonin levels in the brain, in contrast to the prevailing medications like tricyclic compounds, which were not selective, or target-specific and hence had many unwanted side effects. Commenting on this

theme and Prozac's advantage, one psychiatrist put it succinctly when he said: *instead of using a shotgun, you're using a bullet!*

5. The once-a-day dosage of Prozac increased treatment compliance, which was a major advantage. In addition, Eli Lilly's research showed that 75 to 80 percent of depressed patients responded well to Prozac. Increasing the number of patients who are currently not seeking treatment, seek medical help is possible only by increasing awareness of depression and possible treatment among physicians and patients. The prescriber and prescription bases can be widened when you promote the product to primary care physicians (doctors in family practice and internal medicine) and not just psychiatrists. The company decided to promote the drug to primary care physicians and psychiatrists. To achieve this, Lilly planned to develop a comfort level among PCPs in treating depression. PCPs, who are the gatekeepers of medicine, have the potential to drive prescriptions upward. The company, therefore, funded a program wherein key opinion leaders were sent out to large PCP conferences and other medical meetings to share their expert knowledge and experiences of Prozac. Drug reps fanned out to PCP offices across the country to make the sales calls.
6. Lilly also made use of two more channels to optimize its promotion. Sampling to induce trial among new patients and medical journal advertising to sway more doctors towards prescribing Prozac for newly diagnosed patients with depression.
7. Lilly launched a massive direct-to-consumer program to increase awareness of depression as a treatable disorder. This is because depression at the time remained a seriously under-diagnosed and under-treated illness. It was estimated that two out of every three depressed patients did not receive treatment. By targeting those reluctant to seek professional help for their symptoms, the campaign attempted to deal with many people. The campaign's objective was to encourage people suffering from depression to get treatment.

Introduced in 1987, Prozac immediately revolutionized the treatment of depression. By 1996, Prozac had been prescribed to more than 17 million Americans and had achieved $2.36 billion in sales worldwide. It accounted for about 29 percent of Eli Lilly's total revenues. But, then, success brings with it competition. Huge success brings huge competition. That's what happened to Prozac. There were two Prozac-like (SSRI) drugs challenging Lilly's Prozac. In addition, Pfizer's Zoloft had become the second largest-selling antidepressant with $1.7 billion, closely followed by GSK's Paxil with $1. 45 billion in annual sales. These competitive threats spelled urgency for Eli Lilly as its stakes are high in the antidepressant market, with Prozac accounting for nearly a third of the company's total revenues.

Eli Lilly responded to these mounting pressures from competition and the slowing pace of growth by launching a major advertising campaign in print media targeting patients directly, not physicians. The print ad campaign by Leo Burnett Company in Chicago used weather imaging to amplify its message symbolically, such as—dark clouds giving way to bright sunshine—from a Sun that is somewhat evocative of the *happy face* symbol, which urged everyone to *have a nice day* in the 1990s to promote Prozac. This antidepressant treatment symbolized how consumers in the 1990s tried to cure their ills with pills. The company released its print ad campaign in twenty popular magazines and journals, including Family Circle, Good Housekeeping, Sports Illustrated, Cosmopolitan, Men's Health, Newsweek, Time, Parade Magazine, Entertainment Weekly, etc. There was a gender bias toward women's readership in selecting the journals and magazines. Research indicated that women accounted for 60 percent of doctor visits and were twice as likely as men to request a specific brand of medication. There were two main reasons why Lilly chose the print media for its DTC campaign:

1. Firstly, the limitations placed by the US FDA on DTC television ads. Regulations in force at the time prohibited pharmaceutical

companies from drawing an explicit connection between a medical condition and medication. Print ads were not circumscribed by such restrictions and, therefore, a better way for Lilly to convey its message to consumers.

2. Secondly, a print ad gave consumers more time to reflect than a 30-second television spot, which was ideal for Lilly's campaign purposes.

As Mike Grossman, Leo Burnett's Director of Public Relations, explained, Lilly's print campaign had one main communication objective. It had to assist people in their depressed stupor to raise their hands for help. They might not recognize their condition, or know that help is out there. Therefore, the campaign had to overcome the stigma surrounding depression and other mental illnesses. As a result, the advertising copy was carefully crafted to describe the symptoms of depression in a non-threatening way:

So you may have trouble sleeping...feeling unusually sad or irritable...Find it hard to concentrate...lose your appetite...lack energy or have trouble feeling pleasure...

The ads also sought to dispel some of the prevalent misconceptions and fears about depression:

It isn't just feeling down. It's a real illness with real causes...some people think you can just will yourself out of depression... That's not true.

Behind the print ad campaign of Eli Lilly, there was a lot of qualitative consumer research. The company talked to 900 consumers in great depth, spending intensive time with depressed patients seeking treatment. One finding from this research partly explains why depression remained such an under-diagnosed and under-treated illness. Some respondents, who came from a boomer generation, said their parents asked them: *Why don't you pick yourself up?*

Not only the copy, even the visuals resonated with depressed patients who did not seek treatment for their illness earlier. This is because the visual elements in the campaign ads were inspired by patients' illustrations of their feelings about depression and recovery. The campaign intended to connect depressed readers or their family members and friends on an emotional level. The simple yet powerful symbols of darkness and light were developed to be inclusive.

The original ad was a three-page magazine spread that featured sharply contrasting images portraying the darkness experienced by a person suffering from depression and the visual on the second (facing) page showing the light that a patient felt when the illness abated. The first page consisted of a gray cloud on a black background and a copy line saying: *Depression hurts*. The opposite page was a vibrant blue with a highly stylized drawing of a yellow Sun captioned with the campaign's signature line: *Prozac can help*.

There was copy beneath the visuals that described the symptoms of depression in a non-threatening way. The final paragraph encouraged readers to seek medical help if their symptoms matched those described in the ad and closed by stating that: *Prozac has been prescribed to more than 1 million Americans. Chances are someone you know is feeling sunny again because of it. Prozac. Welcome back*.

In the months following the publication of the initial ad, Lilly released two companion ads. Each featured the same text, and all were thematically similar. One of the new ads substituted a broken vase, and a vase holding flowers for the gray cloud and the yellow Sun of the original ad. The other, which ran only in November and December 1997, displayed a limp Christmas tree on one page and a sturdy uptight tree on the opposite page. The creative inspiration for these images came from Lilly's focus groups with depressed patients. The dual metaphorical images of darkness and light accurately expressed to the target audience (depressed patients and their families and friends) what depression and a return to health felt like. Lilly also sought input from doctors and mental health advocacy groups before releasing the original ad to the public.

The DTCA (Direct-to-Consumer-Advertising) campaign encouraged the reader to muse actively over the symptoms. As Gary Mitchell, a professor at the Indiana University of Medical Center, observed, the ad provoked the readers with a question like— You are on Paxil, and you see the Prozac ad and ask yourself, *Why Am I not on that drug?*

The campaign also drew some negative responses from columnists and consumer advocacy groups. The drug companies were creating demand through consumer advertising, which could be a problem, and physicians would prescribe drugs their patients asked for. At the same time, there was praise from many doctors and mental health alliances. They appreciated the campaign's efforts to educate many individuals who suffered, undiagnosed and untreated, from the often debilitating depression.

Prozac's launch and overall marketing effort can only be described as excellent, even unprecedented, because it has become a standard operating procedure for all brands introduced in the CNS (Central Nervous System) therapeutic area. The following table presents important milestones in Prozac's journey.

Table 1.7 Key Milestones in the Development of Prozac: A Timeline

Milestones	Activity
1975	Fluoxetine generic name approved.
1976	Fluoxetine IND submitted to the US FDA, Phase I trial initiated.
1978	Phase II trial initiated.
1979	First indication of anti-depressant effect.
1981	Phase III trials initiated.
1983	NDA submitted to US FDA.
1985	FDA advisory committee unanimously endorsed Fluoxetine.
1986	Fluoxetine (Prozac) was approved and launched in Belgium for the treatment of depression.
1987	Prozac was approved and launched in the United States for the treatment of depression.

Table 1.7 *Contd...*

Milestones	Activity
1992	Annual sales of Prozac reached US $ 1 billion in the United States.
1994	A. New indication approval for Prozac. FDA approved Prozac for the treatment Obsessive Compulsive Disorder (OCD) in the US. B. Prozac attained the name recognition of *Kleenex* and social status of *Spring Water* in the United States, as quoted in a Newsweek article.
1996	Another New indication approval for Prozac. FDA approved Prozac for the treatment of *bulimia nervosa* in the US.
1997	Eli Lilly launched its first-ever print ad campaign for Prozac in about 20 popular magazines in the United States.
1999	Prozac named as one of the Products of the Century by Fortune magazine putting it in the company of Penicillin, Band-Aid, Radio, Television, World Wide Web.
2000	Over 38 million patients have been prescribed Prozac according to estimates.
2001	Prozac's market exclusivity expired in the United States.

Prozac had become trendy with its marketing and set future brand trends. Prozac's marketing strategy had many firsts to its credit. Right from naming the brand to systematic grooming and development of KOLs to become its spokespersons, focusing on PCPs, and listening to depressed patients to understand their perceptions, and built it into a meaningful, memorable DTCA campaign— with all these activities, Eli Lilly had set a standard which was followed and practiced by many pharmaceutical firms even today.

(Source: Adapted from articles—(1)Margaret L. Eaton, Mark Xu, *Developing and Marketing a Blockbuster Drug: Lessons from Eli Lilly's Experience with Prozac*, Harvard Business Publishing Education, February 25, (2) Jeremy Laurance, *Health Check: Science Created Prozac but Marketing Made it Sing*, Independent, February 2, 1999)

CASE

14

How A Fifth-in-Class Drug Became A Top-in-Class Drug in Sales!

The story of Lipitor (Atorvastatin) is also the story of a fifth-in-class drug that became a top-in-lass drug in sales. It has many interesting twists and turns to it. The plot thickens with each twist and turn, and involves a merger of two companies, a co-marketing arrangement, and a hostile acquisition.

On November 3, 1999, Warner-Lambert and American Home Products (AHP) announced an ambitious merger that would create the world's largest pharmaceutical company with combined revenues of $26 billion and a market capitalization of $145 billion. The following day, on November 4, 1999, Pfizer made the largest hostile takeover bid in the history of pharmaceuticals. Pfizer offered a stock transfer offer of $80 billion for Warner-Lambert and finally acquired it for $90.2 billion on February 7, 2000.

Warner-Lambert, founded in the early 1850s, has evolved considerably throughout its history to become one of the largest pharmaceutical companies. The company expanded through many acquisitions and mergers to become an international competitor in many businesses. However, the prescription drug business has always been important to Warner-Lambert, with over 57 percent of sales coming from it. The acquisition of Parke-Davis in 1970 further sharpened Warner-Lambert's focus on the prescription drug business.

Warner-Lambert faced many setbacks in its pharmaceutical business in the early 1990s. The consequent bad press and poor ratings from industry analysts worsened the situation. As a part of its recovery process, the company had cut back its resources on R&D. Ronald Cresswell, chairman of pharmaceutical research at the time, chose to focus his limited resources on a few promising molecules, leaving aside the products in the early stages of development. Fortunately (in retrospect) for the company, one of the chemical compounds retained for development was Atorvastatin (Lipitor).

The Statin Scenario

The discovery of statins, a new therapeutic class, revolutionized the treatment of high cholesterol in the late 1980s. After forty-five years of research, Merck launched the first-ever statin drug Mevacor (lovastatin), in 1987. Close on the heels of Mevacor's launch, entered three more statins, Pravachol (Pravastatin) of Bristol-Myers Squibb, Zocor (Simvastatin) of Merck, and Lescol (Fluvastatin) of Novartis. Lipitor would be the fifth statin. As the tradition goes, the fifth-in-class drug has little chance of succeeding in the market. The following table presents the relative market shares of the four cholesterol-reducing drugs before Lipitor entered the market.

Table 1.8 Cholesterol-Reducing Drugs and Market Shares of Four Statins

Drug Name	Company	Launch Year	Market Share (%)
Mevacor (Lovastatin)	Merck	1987	14
Pravachol (Pravastatin)	Bristol-Myers Squibb	1991	21
Zocor (Simvastatin)	Merck	1992	32
Lescol (Fluvastatin)	Novartis	1994	14

Lipitor's retention of the statin faced severe criticism as it was a fifth statin drug, therefore, a me-too product that would enter an already crowded market dominated by products from some of the most powerful pharmaceutical companies in the world. But, a Phase-I study in 1992 provided a ray of hope for Warner-Lambert that Lipitor could be a powerful cholesterol-reducing agent. A 1994 Phase II study converted that ray of hope into a belief as it showed Lipitor's 60 percent more cholesterol-reducing power over its competitors in the market. With renewed confidence about the differentiability of their product, Warner-Lambert went into Lipitor's Phase III trials. Lipitor is significantly superior to competitors in its ability to reduce cholesterol levels.

Fifth-in-Class to Top-in-Class: Lipitor's Journey

How did Lipitor move from a fifth-in-class market to Top-in-class in sales? Having realized that Lipitor is significantly superior to the competition in its cholesterol-reducing ability, Warner-Lambert was determined to realize the potential of its super statin drug, Lipitor. The company took some very important strategic decisions to make it happen. Here are some of its more significant strategic decisions:

1. Decided to run Phase-III trials with people suffering from familial hypercholesterolemia, a fatal hereditary condition resulting in exceptionally high cholesterol, to get a fast track clearance from the FDA. A small minority of people suffer from this condition, and any competitive statins did not clinically address it. The FDA will consider the drug for fast track clearance (six months compared to the average of 12 months), if it treats a serious, or life-threatening condition, or addresses an unmet need. The trial results justified a fast track clearance, and the FDA approved Lipitor within six months of the New Drug Application (NDA).
2. Another significant decision was to conduct head-to-head clinical trials against the leading competing statins. The marketing group at Warner-Lambert requested this. This tactic is rarely followed in the drug industry because, if the new product fails to show significant superiority to competitors, it would be very difficult to persuade physicians to switch their patients to the new drug. Of course, it would be an extremely desirable asset if the drug is superior to the competition.

Fortunately for the company, Lipitor was superior to all other statins in the market. In the head-to-head trials, Lipitor reduced elevated cholesterol by 40 to 60 percent across the full dose range (10 mg to 80 mg) and reduced triglycerides by 19 to 40 percent. The best-selling competitive cholesterol reducer, Zocor of Merck, decreased LDL cholesterol by only about 40 percent.

3. Ronald Cresswell's initiative of integrating regulatory affairs and clinical research into the R&D organization to improve the documentation process was another useful strategic decision. He has also involved the marketing earlier in the new product development process. This initiative too helped the company as it brought both R&D and marketing on the same page regarding Lipitor's potential long before its approval.
4. In addition, Warner-Lambert developed a compensation plan uncapping performance incentives, which enabled successful performers to earn huge amounts and raise the salesforce morale significantly.

Marketing Lipitor

Warner-Lambert faced many serious challenges in bringing Lipitor to the market. The first challenge is that it is the fifth statin to enter the market. Although proven superior in clinical trials compared to all other statins in the market, Lipitor was seen as a 'me-too' drug by patients, physicians, and payers. To top it, the incumbents such as Merck and Bristol-Myers Squibb had proven products in the market. The competitors also enjoyed strong relationships with key opinion leaders, such as cardiologists. And they all had experienced sales forces— larger than Warner-Lambert. So how could a smaller company, Warner-Lambert fight the dominant competitors and grab a respectable market share?

A successful launch of Lipitor is a marketing imperative. The first six months after a drug launch are crucial for its success. The initial adoption rate of the drug by physicians can often make, or break a new product. The most important challenge of all is to launch Lipitor effectively. The company brainstormed and arrived at a launch strategy. The key elements of Lipitor's launch strategy were:

1. *Marketing Alliance with Pfizer:* Warner-Lambert decided on a *saturation* approach to market Lipitor. The market for cholesterol-reducing drugs had several untreated patients and physicians who were largely content with the therapeutic solution already available. They were not looking for new therapies. By pursuing a *saturation* strategy, the company wanted to contact as many physicians as possible, including the universe of US cardiologists at the time. The company needs many sales representatives to achieve this broad coverage of physicians. Its existing salesforce is not adequate. Recruiting such a large sales force for marketing one product did not make economic sense. The alternative? Co-marketing. Creating a marketing alliance with a reputed pharmaceutical company that does not have conflicting interests in product promotion. Anthony Wild, Warner-Lambert pharmaceutical sector vice president at the time, explained the need for the salesforce augmentation best when he said: *The more soldiers you have out there, the more guns, the more likely you are to achieve your ends*.

   Therefore, the company decided that a partnership was necessary to address its constrained sales and marketing resources and narrowed its search for marketing partners to two— Hoffman-La Roche and Pfizer. Its choice of Pfizer as a marketing partner was more a matter of chance. At one point in the negotiation, a Warner-Lambert fax intended for Hoffman-La Roche accidentally ended up in a Pfizer fax machine. The unintended fax helped persuade Pfizer to make a great offer to get the Lipitor deal. Finally, Warner-Lambert chose Pfizer as its marketing partner because of its marketing experience, relationships with cardiologists, its track record of successful product launches. The highlights of the Lipitor Marketing alliance with Pfizer were:

- Pfizer paid $205 million in upfront money and milestone payments for the rights to sell Lipitor. Pfizer also agreed to split all future product expenses, including advertising, promotion, sampling, and sales force.
- Furthermore, Pfizer agreed to pay for half of any ongoing and planned clinical trials, which were more than a hundred and involved 100,000 patients.
- In return, Pfizer would receive variable payments based on sales targets established in the agreement. Pfizer has been receiving about 48 percent of net sales.

2. *Product Positioning of Lipitor:* Lipitor was positioned as a superior cholesterol-reducing drug first and foremost. The head-to-head clinical trials proved its efficacy as the most potent statin in the market in reducing elevated total cholesterol, LDL cholesterol, and triglycerides over a range of comparable doses.

   Lipitor was the first drug approved for reducing triglycerides and the more common LDL cholesterol making it an ideal drug for a broad range of points. Although Pravachol (Bristol-Myers Squibb) and Zocor (Merck) are also effective in lowering high triglycerides, neither Bristol-Myers Squibb nor Merck possessed the *triglyceride indication* at the time of Lipitor launch.

   Ease of use was another important positioning message Lipitor established in the mind of the physicians. Physicians found it difficult to determine a patient's optimal dose with other available statins. Instead, they had to select a starting dose, retest the patient's cholesterol after using the drug, adjust the dose, and repeat the cycle until they identified the proper dose. Fortunately for Lipitor, 72 percent of patients reach the target LDL cholesterol goal at the starting dose of 10-milligram dose, thereby eliminating the need for the cumbersome procedure of testing, adjusting, and retesting.

3. *Lipitor's Value Positioning: Pricing:* Lipitor achieved the position of the most value-for-money with its moderate pricing. Warner-

Lambert made the already-convincing-Lipitor value proposition even better with its pricing strategy. Lipitor was positioned as the product with therapeutic superiority and ease of use, yet priced lower than the market-leading competitors. The following table presents the comparative prices of leading statin brands in the US in 1997.

Table 1.9 Average Prescription Prices of Statin Drugs in the US in 1997

Statin Brand / Company	Average Price US $
1. Mevacor / Merck	125
2. Zocor / Merck	95
3. Pravachol / Bristol-Myers Squibb	93
4. Lipitor / Warner-Lambert	84

4. *Lipitor: Promotional Tactics:* Lipitor had put in a massive pre-launch effort. Its pre-launch tactics included:

   A. Even before launching Lipitor, Warner-Lambert launched a national cholesterol education program in conjunction with American Heart Association (AHA) to educate patients and physicians that cholesterol needed to be treated more aggressively than it was; they needed to *go for the goal* established in the guidelines set by the national cholesterol education program. The campaign positioned Lipitor as the drug best suited for achieving these targets.

   B. In addition, Lipitor made good use of its pre-market comparative efficacy data by publicizing it in medical journals and at major medical conventions.

   C. The company recruited key opinion leaders (KOLs) to use free samples immediately after Lipitor was approved but before it was formally launched.

   D. All these pre-marketing efforts resulted in Lipitor achieving 3 percent of all new cholesterol-lowering prescriptions.

   E. The combined salesforce of Warner-Lambert and Pfizer, numbering 2,200, was the largest to promote a statin brand in the US. They targeted about 91,000 key prescribers—

physicians within the cardiology area, interns, and general and family practitioners who were known prescribers of cholesterol-lowering drugs.

F. Lipitor has achieved a 29 percent share of voice, the highest among all statin drugs in the market in the launch year.

G. The combined salesforce of Warner-Lambert and Pfizer implemented a very aggressive e-sampling program. They distributed 7.3 million samples of Lipitor to physicians in the first year of launch.

H. The company had its moment of luck. The year of Lipitor's launch was also the year when FDA allowed prescription drug advertising, targeting consumers. Direct-to-consumer-advertising (DTCA) began in 1997. Warner-Lambert benefited from this significantly. The company spent millions of dollars on DTCA urging patients to *Know Your Numbers,* and then showing patients how Lipitor helped them get their cholesterol numbers below guidelines goals.

I. Pfizer acquired Warner-Lambert by a hostile takeover in 2000 and gained total control of Lipitor.

J. Pfizer conducted focus groups with doctors and unearthed key selling points its competitors missed. The company found that doctors were scared of the dosages of statins. This helped significantly in highlighting the simplicity of Lipitor's dosage.

K. Lipitor has achieved wide insurance coverage and Medicare eligibility, improving its access considerably.

L. Pfizer continued research on Lipitor and conducted more than 400 clinical studies, including more than 80,000 patients costing about a billion dollars. These studies have shown how Lipitor helped patients with heart problems and associated risks such as stroke and heart attacks.

Success Right From the Start!

Lipitor has been a spectacular success right from the start. First synthesized by Dr. Bruce Roth, a chemist at Warner-Lambert, in 1982,

Lipitor entered the market with FDA approval in 1997 as a fifth-in-class statin drug. Since then, Lipitor has never looked back. Nicknamed, *Turbostatin* for its superior cholesterol-reducing ability, Lipitor passed the coveted $1 billion in the launch year itself. Within three years, Lipitor became the largest-selling statin drug and the first-ever prescription drug to pass the $12 billion mark in annual sales. Furthermore, Lipitor became the largest-selling prescription drug in history, with lifetime sales of $140.75 billion from its launch till its patent expired in 2012. Even after five years after losing its market exclusivity, Lipitor continues to be a valuable asset to Pfizer, with annual sales of $0.9 billion in 2017.

Lipitor's *How* Wins Over Mevacor's *Where*!

The key to Lipitor's unprecedented success was its basic strategic approach. While the pioneer among statins— Mevacor, chose the position of *Where to compete*, Lipitor, a late entrant, and a fifth-in-class drug chose *How to compete*. The difference between the positions— *Where* and *How* was crucial. By choosing the *Where* position, Mevacor decided rightly for a pioneer in defining the market. By definition, defining the market means creating the market for a particular product class, and that would also pave the way for competition to enter. While focusing on where to compete was essential, it should not have focused exclusively on *where* to compete. When it launched Mevacor, Merck was not ready with all its vital clinical research data. The company was still conducting its 4-S Study (The Scandinavian Simvastatin in Survival Study). Merck did not initially spend adequate time and effort to educate the doctors and the public about its product and what it could do to improve their heart health. Merck rushed its Mevacor into the market and began its disease awareness and education campaign.

Pfizer chose an altogether different strategy. The strategy of *How* to compete. As a late entrant into the statin market, Pfizer focused on reaching more doctors and gaining approval for prescribing Lipitor.

The key question is—How to make Lipitor communication more effective? The company's head-to-head trials with its major competitors were a part of the *How* to strategy. More importantly, Warner-Lambert was ready with its clinical data to establish Lipitor's significant superiority over its competitors before it launched Lipitor. It had also trained its sales force adequately on how to convert doctors prescribing other statins to prescribing Lipitor.

Brilliant Campaign, Frayed Execution

Pfizer launched a brilliant Direct-to-consumer (DTC) advertising campaign for Lipitor just as the first generics of Simvastatin (Zocor) were entering the market. The company released a full week of full-color, full-page advertisements in the New York Times in June 2006. The objective was to protect Lipitor prescriptions from being substituted with Simvastatin generics.

The advertising campaign featured Robert Jarvik, the medical investigator-cum-entrepreneur credited with the invention of the *Jarvik Artificial Heart*. The advertisements showed Jarvik rowing a boat. In the advertisements towards the close, Jarvik looking straight into the camera, says: *I take Lipitor. For me, there is no substitute.* The Jarvik— Lipitor advertisements taught patients to be cautious about the probable generic substitution for Lipitor by physicians, pharmacists, and insurers.

The campaign revolved around authenticity. For the first time, the celebrity endorser was a real doctor, not an actor who played the doctor's role in a prescription drug campaign. The campaign became highly visible and, at the same time, highly controversial. Choosing Jarvik as the celebrity brand ambassador for Lipitor boomeranged. Because Robert Jarvik was not a cardiologist, he never completed a residency program, although he completed an undergraduate course in medicine from an offshore medical school. As a result, he was not licensed to prescribe and practice. Critics also argued that Jarvik claimed credit for inventing the artificial heart, but the concept and technology behind the invention predated his work. Furthermore, a middle-aged rower from Seattle, Dennis Williams, who bore a close resemblance to Jarvik, announced that he had served as Jarvik's body double in the video shoot of the Lipitor that showed Jarvik rowing the boat. Jarvik's admission later that he did not use Lipitor until after he had been hired as a Pfizer spokesperson implied that his advertising message of Lipitor being responsible for his cardiovascular health was untrue.

All these had a very adverse impact on the credibility ty of the campaign. Later, Pfizer replaced the rowing advertisement with Jarvik jogging with his son. But, these revelations were intensely damaging for a marketing campaign based on the importance of authenticity. Later in 2007, there was a congressional hearing where the portrayal of Jarvik as a spokesperson and the positioning of Lipitor as superior to generic statins were explicitly linked in.

Pfizer withdrew Jarvik from the Lipitor advertisements but stayed on with its campaign stating that *Lipitor is Lipitor*, with the underlying message of inimitableness.

Whistle Blowing Case

Dr. Jesse Polansky, former director of outcomes management strategy at Pfizer, who was responsible for reviewing some of the marketing materials for Lipitor and other products, filed a lawsuit against Pfizer regarding the unethical marketing practices of Lipitor, seeking compensation as a whistleblower. His main allegations against the company were:

- Pfizer gave unrestricted education grants. These Grants were a part of the marketing plans of Lipitor, with a clear objective of creating a medical platform supporting Lipitor's new positioning.
- Pfizer wanted to extend Lipitor use beyond the indications found on the table by targeting people at moderate risk of developing heart disease or having a heart attack. People with moderate risk did not need Lipitor therapy.

- Pfizer programs included deliberate misinformation promoting the idea that kidney-disease patients may need statin treatment.

Here is what Pfizer said in response to all the allegations:

We believe this case has no merit. Furthermore, after reviewing the allegations in the complaint, the government declined to intervene in their action. Pfizer does not condone the off-label promotion of one of its products. We believe our sales and marketing practices are solely based on our prescription information approved by the FDA.

Defending Against Generics

Pfizer implemented a raft of initiatives to stem Lipitor's loss of market share and revenue, its most valuable asset to generic rivals, before its patent expiry. The US accounted for around 55 percent of Lipitor's $10.7 bill on worldwide sales. In addition, Pfizer made significant efforts to capitalize on brand loyalty, and the emotional attachment of patients and prescribers to Lipitor, which is unusual in prescription drug marketing. Pfizer took several measures to encourage prescribers and patients to stay with the Lipitor brand even when generics are available.

Some of the more important initiatives of Pfizer are:

- Pfizer signed discounted deals with Pharmacy Benefit Managers (PBMs) and health insurers, including reduced copays for Lipitor.
- Pfizer also took an unusual step of setting up its own mail-order service to supply Lipitor to patients who have been taking Lipitor for years, want to stay with Lipitor, and are reluctant to switch to generics.
- Pfizer Licensed a generic version (authorized generic) of Lipitor to Watson pharmaceuticals.

Pfizer's initiatives to minimize the generic loss have helped the copay significantly. Even after six years of its patent expiry, Lipitor achieved sales of $0.9 billion in 2017. Lipitor is a classic example of launch excellence and marketing excellence.

Lessons

Christopher Bowe identified three important lessons from Lipitor's success that are valuable to all pharmaceutical marketers in his Harvard Business Review article, *Say farewell to Lipitor, but don't forget its lessons* on November 18, 2011. First, he very aptly observed that getting bigger through mega-mergers has not proven to make big Pharma accomplish better at their core task of producing innovative products. Pfizer's case (despite Lipitor's unprecedented success) validates that. Here are the Lessons:

1. *Resist the lure of strategies that depend on a single source of power.* Pfizer was a different company when the acquisition bug bit it in 1999. It was smaller but intensely aspirational and obsessed with getting even with the bigger Merck, the industry leader at the time. Pfizer's primary motivation for acquiring Warner-Lambert, the owner of Lipitor and with whom it had a co-marketing alliance, is to gain total control and ownership of Lipitor and become bigger. A decade later, in retrospect, that motive seems to have been based more on hubris than on setting the company on a sustainable path to continued success.
2. *When a strategic distraction occurs, don't add more distractions.* Lipitor's spectacular success and the Warner-Lambert acquisition seem to be a one-trick pony with limited prospects for organic growth. To fuel further growth, Pfizer engineered another large-scale merger with Pharmacia in 2003, to gain control of Celebrex. This anti-arthritic drug was thought to be very promising at the time. Later in 2009, Pfizer acquired Wyeth to form the world's premier biopharmaceutical company. All these acquisitions caused disruption and distraction as Pfizer struggled to integrate them.
3. *Acquisitions should fund innovation, not replace it.* All the oceans of money that Lipitor generated over its lifetime (over

$131 billion) did not help to keep the Pfizer share price stable over the years. The company's share peaked in June 2000, five months after the Warner-Lambert deal was announced. In 2011, Pfizer's price fell 60 percent below its historic peak, and the shareholder value suffered. The company could not protect its share price from a broad decline and stagnation, despite enormous cash generation that fueled dividends and other returns.

Pfizer, due to its heavy dependence on one drug for revenues and beset with distracting acquisitions, was unable to innovate on its own. The pharmaceutical industry's key rationale for high prices for branded drugs is that they fund innovation, not acquisitions. Innovation brings value, but acquisitions do not necessarily so.

(Source: Adapted from articles—1. It took a brilliant marketing campaign to create the best-selling drug of all time, businessinsider.com, 2. Christopher Bowe, Say farewell to Lipitor, but don't forget its lessons, Harvard Business Review, November 18, 2011, hbr.org, 3. Lipitor: How far should Pfizer push the pill, ICMR (IBS Center for Management Research) Case study)

Positioning Based on Marketing-Mix Variables

Pharma marketers can create a distinct positioning for their brand by differentiating any element of their marketing mix from the competition to make it memorable. For example, the size and quality of a field force can give a brand an important and sustainable edge. Two companies that used field force as a distinct competitive advantage are:

- Merck Sharp and Dohme (MSD) used this for Vasotec (enalapril maleate).
- Glaxo expanded its field force coverage through a co-marketing alliance with Roche when it launched Zantac (ranitidine hydrochloride), in the US.
- Earlier, Marion (Sanofi, now) capitalized on a talented sales force and marketed in-licensed good products from other companies in the US.
- In addition, pharmaceutical companies in the US mainly pursue positioning strategies in hospital and managed healthcare markets, using differentiated services like custom labeling, instant delivery, and custom packaging.

Here are two cases illustrating how two pharmaceutical companies used two marketing mix elements to differentiate their brands and won. One is the case of Rocephin, where Roche used communication as a differentiator, and the other is Zithromax, where Pfizer used packaging to differentiate its brand.

CASE

15

Rocephin Stands Out in a Crowded Market!

Hoffman La Roche, the Swiss drug major, launched its broad-spectrum injectable antibiotic in the United States in 1993. The injectable antibiotic market was indeed crowded at the time. Injectable antibiotics are used mainly in hospitals to treat serious and life-threatening conditions. The ability to kill the invading germs or the killing power was the main criterion for selecting the drug for hospitals and physicians. Almost all the competing brands of injectable antibiotics claimed that their brands were the most potent killer antibiotics. Not only was the market crowded, but also the messaging.

Rocephin had a tough challenge, as a new entrant would. How to stand out in the crowded segment of antibiotic injectables? The brand, Rocephin, however, had a distinct advantage. It had a very convenient once-daily dosage, whereas all the other brands had to be given twice daily. Of course, a once-daily dosage is a tremendous advantage. But, the physicians at the time did not think so.

On the contrary, they thought a once-daily dosage was a great disadvantage. Surprising as it may seem, the physicians were apprehensive that despite the substantial evidence confirming the efficacy of Rocephin, its effects might taper off, reducing the antibacterial power over twenty-four hours before the next dose, leaving patients vulnerable to toxic pathogens. The hospitals, too, might become vulnerable and become a target of costly lawsuits.

After thoroughly researching the advertising and messaging practices of competing brands, the brand team of Rocephin observed that all the competitors were harping on their respective 'kill powers' and often showing images of scary, open, infected wounds and blown-up microscopic pathogens. So the Rocephin team decided to follow a different route that would give them a distinct identity in the crowded market. That would make Rocephin stand out.

Instead of engaging in a head-to-head competition highlighting Rocephin's power to kill bacteria, the team focused on what the hospitals and physicians were looking for. *Better outcomes. Quickly and safely discharging the patients who recovered completely from the serious conditions.* In other words, *Wellness On* is getting better, Rapid recovery from infections. The communication, too, was simple, direct, and straightforward. For example, the advertisement shows an image of an apple, denoting the simple yet powerful folksy adage that *an apple a day keeps the doctor away*.

It's simplicity at its best. There was no need for any rational argument, as it resonated with patients, physicians, the hospital staff, and the payers.

Rocephin became a blockbuster and passed the $2.8 billion mark in sales in 2005, the year of its patent expiry. Understandably, generics eroded 55 percent of its market by 2007.

Lessons

The case of Rocephin is a classic example of how to create a distinct brand identity in a crowded marketplace.

Rocephin's communication strategy focused on what customers want and not on what the brand is and brand does. It focused on the outcomes such as healthy recovery, safe discharge from the hospital, and wellness.

As Vince Parry, the thought leader of healthcare advertising strategies, says in his insightful book, *Identity crisis,* Brand identity is a distinguishing set of essential values, or ideas of a product, company, or service perceived by customers.

Rocephin's brand communication was the essence of simplicity. It resonated with all the stakeholders that matter. Rocephin, as a result, owned 'wellness' and not serious problems like competition.

(Source: Adapted from Vince Parry's book *Identity Crisis: Healthcare Branding's Hidden Problems and Proven Strategies to Solve Them)*

CASE

16

The Z-Pak: Packaging As A Differentiator!

Launched in 1991 in the US, Abbott's Biaxin (clarithromycin) was in a leading position when Pfizer launched its antibiotic brand, Zithromax (azithromycin), a year later in 1992.

Clinical evidence showed that Biaxin had superior efficacy but required twenty doses, making adherence to therapy challenging. In comparison, Pfizer's Zithromax required only five doses to complete the course of treatment.

Pfizer accentuated this difference in dosage regimen with innovative packing and introduced the Z-Pak. The Z-Pak is an easy-to-use cardboard box that provides detailed and clear dosing instructions when flipped open. It was unique and easy to carry, and included because of its innovative design, some communication to patients regarding the cost, the importance of completing the full regimen, competitive claims, and further instructions, which a traditional bottle pack cannot provide.

The Z-Pak offered one more advantage, as indicated by patient research. As patients would get a pill bottle with only six Zithromax tablets, the bottle felt fairly empty, with tablets rattling around in the big bottle. As a result, the patients felt they were not getting their money's worth as they were more accustomed to a pill bottle that was mostly full rather than mostly empty. The Z-Pak resolved the impression that Zithromax patients were not getting their money's worth with its simple, innovative Z-Pak that convinced them about its convenient dosage regimen. Finally, Zithromax gained market leadership in the antibiotic space with its Z-Pak!

(Source: Adapted from the book, Brand Plan Rx: The Marketer's Guide to Building a Thriving health and Wellness Brand, by Markus Saba & Hilary GentileBrightWing Media, 2021)

Positioning by *Price*

The price positioning is placing a price on a product or service within a certain price range, indicating where it sits (position) in relation to its competition in customers' minds.

When you align pricing and positioning, the *price* can be an important element of your positioning strategy. For example, if you sell a luxury product or service, you need to position your product at the high end of the market, reflecting a premium position for your brand. On the contrary, if you want to offer value for money, your pricing will have to reflect its affordability position. Of course, you should consider several aspects, such as your marketing objectives (penetrating the market or skimming the cream of the market), profitability, available competitive spaces, and many more when you want to use pricing as a positioning strategy.

The following two cases show how two pharma companies— a global pharma major for an innovative prescription drug brand and a branded generic drug firm in India (for their entire product mix) have used pricing as a strategy and won.

CASE

17

How Glaxo Won the Anti-Ulcer Market!

Glaxo (GSK now), the British pharmaceutical giant, developed ranitidine and launched it under the brand name Zantac in many countries. SKF's (GSK now) Tagamet was reigning supreme in the anti-ulcer market with annual sales of over US $950 million and was aiming to become the first-ever prescription drug to cross the US $1 billion in annual sales. However, Zantac of Glaxo shattered all those dreams, for it was Zantac that became the first-ever prescription drug to pass the US $1 billion mark.

How did Glaxo win with Zantac? First, Glaxo obtained a higher price for Zantac than Tagamet of SKF, which was the first of H2 antagonists and the market leader, using a skim-the-cream strategy to recover the high R&D investment faster. Then, to reinforce the communications cue of quality and superiority that the relatively high priced Zantac offered, Glaxo launched a prestige campaign and differentiated their anti-ulcer drug Zantac by positioning it as a superior product, a Super Tagamet in the doctors' minds.

In India, too, Glaxo followed the skimming strategy for their Zinetec brand of ranitidine when they launched it in 1986. The company priced it very high, almost one hundred percent above many competitors' prices.

The company very aggressively pursued a promotional strategy to desensitize the customers to the high price and reinforce the quality cues offered by the high price. These included seminars, lecture sessions for doctors in class I towns and metro-cities, by eminent gastroenterologists from all over the world, persuasion by a team of highly proficient and well-trained medical representatives, samples, gifts, an attractive premium-looking pack and a differentiated product in the form of a specially coated tablet (all other formulations were plain tablets). Consequently, Glaxo achieved brand leadership for Zinetec in the very first year of its introduction.

Later, the company had to drastically reduce the price of Zinetec, consequent to the DPCO 1987, to almost half its introductory price. The company followed a penetration strategy (it had virtually no choice) and made the most of it by making customers perceive it as enhanced value for their money.

The price reduction, however, did not affect the quality image of the product since the doctors and pharmacists were aware that the price reduction was not voluntary but a result of a government order (DPCO 1987).

By following a skimming strategy for their Zinetec in India, Glaxo recovered the development costs faster and could afford the heavy promotional expenditure in establishing it as a market leader. When the company was forced to reduce the price of Zinetec, Glaxo valiantly pursued an aggressive market growth strategy, thereby increasing its sales volume considerably. The result was a formidable leadership position in the Indian anti-ulcer market with over 20 percent market share, growing at an impressive 18 percent (1988).

CASE

18

Mankind Pharma Storms into Indian Pharmaceutical Market with its Penetrative Pricing!

When the entire pharmaceutical industry in India is complaining about drug price control, Mankind Pharma, like a true contrarian, followed a penetrative pricing strategy. Penetrative pricing is a marketing strategy used by businesses worldwide to attract customers to a new product or service. However, using it as a strategy for the whole company's pricing policy or philosophy is not seen in the pharmaceutical industry. In the retail business, Walmart and Costco, the supermarket giants in the US, followed the policy of penetrative pricing and achieved leadership positions. No pharmaceutical company has used a penetrative pricing strategy across the board. What is Mankind's pricing strategy? To offer the patients (consumers) all their products at lower prices — 30 to 40 percent lower than the major players in the industry.

The result? Mankind Pharma today has reached the top of the pharmaceutical league table in India with the maximum number of prescriptions to its credit. In addition, the company currently occupies the first rank in prescriptions generated and fourth in sales value for 2022 in the Indian pharmaceutical industry. An unprecedented achievement indeed!

Corporate Positioning

As early as 1986, Philip Kotler suggested that although everyone in marketing worldwide focuses on positioning their products, corporate positioning plays an important role. This is because corporate positioning creates and reinforces a favorable overall position for a pharmaceutical company that is important for its stakeholders.

1. *Prescribers and Patients*: A favorable company image can help Pharma build credibility and trust among physicians and patients, its main stakeholders, and serve as a risk reduction mechanism. Many pharmaceutical companies recognize the importance of developing and building a positive relationship for the long term. For example, in Italy, there was a perceived trend of unethical marketing practices of 'buying' doctors in the 1980s. As a result, Glaxo launched a program involving 30,000 key physicians to strengthen Glaxo's relationship with doctors in Italy to correct the course and bring marketing back on the scientific track.
2. *Stockmarket*: The company's global image is also an important factor on which the stock market assesses the value of a company's stock. A favorable image can be crucial in potential mergers, capital expansion, and takeovers.
3. *Government and Regulatory Agencies*: A positive image of the company can significantly help get speedy regulatory approvals.
4. *Special Interest Groups*: A favorable corporate image will help avoid or preempt the actions of unions and consumer organizations.
5. *Employees*: The positive image created by corporate positioning, using the information on the company's experience, safety record, image as an innovator, leadership position in therapeutic categories, corporate responsibility activities, and commitment to basic research will be of immense help in attracting and retaining talent and improve employee loyalty.

Multiple Segment Positioning

While targeting multiple segments for one's brand may be tempting as it offers a wider scope, conceptually speaking, in practice, such an approach may involve the risk of losing out in all segments. At the same time, concentrating only on one segment means, in effect, throwing away a certain portion of sales. In such a situation, one may use different product forms to cater to the different segments simultaneously, like Ciba-Geigy (Novartis, now) did with their non-steroidal anti-inflammatory brand, Voltaren (diclofenac).

Positioning by Changing the Frame of Reference

How do you position your product if there are no perceptible gaps in the market as defined currently? There is one possibility. It may be possible to alter the map and thus create new opportunities. For example, you may introduce a new attribute and make it salient for the target market (or at least a segment of the target market). Here are two examples of how two big pharma companies did it:

- Buspar, from Bristol-Myers, may have succeeded in doing this in the anti-anxiety drug market. Buspar does not interact with alcohol and is not a controlled substance, so it aimed to create a new segment in converting some anxiety patients from reliance on acute therapy to chronic therapy.
- Tenormin from ICI (AstraZeneca, now) in France introduced the advantage of hydro-solubility in Beta-blockers and succeeded in making this attribute important in that market.

Moving the Competition

Alternatively, you can change the brand's perception in the direction of the ideal product by redirecting competitive brands away from the ideal position. However, you cannot openly denigrate the competition as it may lead to a backlash. Still, it is possible to bring the weaknesses of competing brands to the target audience's notice and ease competition away from the ideal point. Similarly, competitive products can be contrasted to one's product to establish the distinct cases in which the various products should be considered ideal.

Introducing a Fighter (Second) Brand to Defend Your Position

How do you defend your brand when faced with the threat of a new entrant or competitor repositioning his brand against your brand? Innovator brands often face this situation when their product patents expire, and when generic brands enter the market with price as a significant differentiator. So the dilemma before the innovator drug firms is—should they reduce their price and reposition their brand towards the competition on the price dimension, and if so, by how much?

Alternatively, should they launch a brand (generic) to fight the new branded generics on their terms to keep them away from their original brand? The fighter brand (your second brand) then competes with new generic entrants, while the original brand can maintain its profitable pricing position, perhaps with some sacrifice of volume. It is important to position your fighter brand near the competing generics but further away than the main brand to prevent other generic brands from stealing share from the main brand. Here are two examples showing how two pharma majors have used the fighter brand approach to protect their main brand's position against the onslaught of generic brands.

- When Ciba-Geigy's (Novartis, now) Voltaren (diclofenac) patent ran out in France, the company launched a branded generic, Voldar (diclofenac), through Zyma, a company controlled by Ciba-Geigy to protect Voltaren.
- Similarly, SmithKline Beecham (GlaxoSmithKline, now) launched a branded generic to protect Tagamet (cimetidine) when its patent expired.

Positioning at A Corporate Strategy Level

Although not practiced often, it is possible to position a company by differentiating it at a corporate strategy level. From the start, the company will differentiate itself from the rest in all key elements of its strategy. The following case shows how two companies in the Indian pharmaceutical industry chose two different strategic routes and achieved significant success.

CASE

19

Strategy as A Differentiator: A Tale of Two Companies!

Much before Marty Neumeier defined *differentiation* as zagging when your competitors zig in his 2006 best-selling book, *Zag*, two companies in the Indian pharmaceutical industry zagged while the competitors were zigging. But that is taking a different route. A road less traveled, or not traveled.

The two companies started their operations at two different periods with an interval of eleven years between them and at two different places, one in a metro city in eastern India and the other in a town in northern India. Both have been extremely successful and have grown at breakneck speed since their inception year after year, and are among the top five pharma companies in India today. The two companies have one thing in common and that is they followed a differentiation strategy right from the beginning.

The Case of Sun Pharma

The first company, Sun Pharma, started its operations in 1984 in Calcutta City. The company's focus right from its inception was on chronic therapy areas such as psychiatry, neurology, and cardiology. Sun Pharma was not the first company to enter these chronic therapy areas as a strategy. Torrent was. Sun Pharma was the second company. Torrent somehow could not stay focused, whereas Sun Pharma stayed the course and reinforced its specialty focus strategy unflinchingly and unwaveringly. While the rest of the industry has been actively pursuing the big molecules, Sun Pharma chose specialty therapeutic areas such as psychiatry, neurology, and cardiology, indicating its strategic foresight. The reasons why the company focused on these are:

1. The cash value of a single prescription in the chronic therapy area is very high.
2. The Cost of entry is not high as the number of specialty prescribers in each segment is considerably low. The marketing costs to cover these customers are likely to be relatively low as they need a smaller sales force.
3. The lifetime value of a single important super specialty prescriber is huge.

This may be common knowledge today, but in the early 1990s, no other company paid the kind of attention to them as Sun Pharma did. Sun Pharma is the first company to structure its marketing operations around one or two related chronic therapy areas with a laser-sharp focus. It became the first company to have a full-fledged strategic business unit, Synergy (which has grown today to three SBUs), focusing on CNS therapy area to cater to every therapeutic need of psychiatrists and neurologists. Likewise, the company has carved out different SBUs for other chronic therapy areas such as cardiology, diabetes, rheumatology, oncology, etc. With every acquisition the company made to gain access to markets, products, and customers, the company also created a stand-alone SBU to cater to as many as twenty-two specialty therapeutic areas today.

The strategic differentiation did not end with taking a different route. In addition, the company made several winning moves that were significantly different and mastered the art and science of Customer Relationship Management (CRM) in a very organized and systematic manner.

No other company has done that with the focus Sun Pharma has demonstrated in carving out dedicated SBUs to cater to different therapeutic areas and prescriber segments. That's why Sun Pharma has become an undisputed leader in prescriptions and, consequently, revenues generated in many specialty segments such as psychiatry, Neurology, and cardiology. As a result, it is among the top two or three in every segment of its choice.

The company has become the largest pharmaceutical company in India, pushing the earlier leaders behind. Sun Pharma has pursued a similar focused strategy in international markets to emerge as a leading fully integrated international specialty pharma company by sowing the seeds in 1990. As a result, Sun Pharma has achieved the distinction of becoming the fourth largest generics player globally today.

The Case of Mankind Pharma

Eleven years later, in the town of Meerut in the state of Uttar Pradesh, Mankind Pharma started its operations in 1995 with a capital of ₹ 5 million.

Mankind followed a different path as an entry strategy. It selected relatively under-served or unserved markets like small towns, and physicians not fully covered by the rest of the companies and instantly impacted the customers. In addition, it has selected a mass marketing strategy to expand its product portfolio quickly to cover all major molecules and therapeutic segments. Its pricing strategy, too, was different. While it almost became customary to follow competitor-parity in pricing their products for most of the companies in a highly price-controlled market, Mankind priced its products lower, making them more affordable, and this move was appealing to all stakeholders in the pharma industry, including physicians, patients, and general public.

The company also followed some distinctly different strategic and tactical moves, such as:

1. Highly incentivizing performance that is based on growth rather than giving their sales force sales targets or quotas, which has been the industry practice

2. Incentivizing the trade for making the products available to gain their support
3. Covering the universe of the doctors rather than the select few like other pharma companies and following a strategy of reach and frequency model with frequent but not very expensive gifts as brand reminders
4. Focusing on training and development of the sales force to increase their capabilities and confidence

After reaching a critical mass, the company started expanding its customer coverage and therapeutic coverage and created separate marketing units to achieve focus in a multi-specialty marketing environment. As a result, Mankind Pharma has moved up to the coveted fourth position in the Indian pharmaceutical industry today (2022).

The Nuts and Bolts of Brand Positioning

Let us now get to the nuts and bolts of positioning. How can we position our brand differently from the competition in the customer's mind? What makes an ideal positioning for your brand? An aspirational positioning built on deep customer insights and market understanding, differentiated from the competition.

Brand positioning is built on three foundational building blocks—Premise, Promise, and Proof construct, say Markus Saba, and Hilary Gentile, the authors of Brand plan Rx.

- The *Premise* is the insight, unmet need, or a pain point unaddressed in the market.
- The *Promise* is the benefit or solution your brand offers to solve the problem.
- The *Proof* is the reason to believe. It is the evidence, the data, and the key information.

Using this framework, the authors give an example of how it is applied to Nexium (esomeprazole), the antiulcerant drug developed by AstraZeneca.

- Premise: Pain and discomfort from gastroesophageal reflux disease (GERD) may also be damaging the lining of your esophagus
- Promise: Healing purple pill (you not only feel better, you are better)
- Proof: Healing data

You must get all your team members in marketing, sales, medical, customer experience, regulatory, legal, manufacturing, and R&D to be on the same page to have a clear understanding of the positioning. Everybody in your organization should think of healing when they think of Nexium.

Although your positioning statement for Nexium is for internal use, your brand's Premise, Promise, and Proof should resonate with your target patients and physicians. They, too, should think of healing when they think of Nexium.

Brand Positioning Statement

Relationships between customers and brands are increasingly becoming more complex. As a result, brand loyalty has become as fragile as a bubble, particularly in the pharmaceutical industry. Therefore, pharma marketers must do a lot of groundwork to understand the customers' needs for each brand and refine their positioning strategies to achieve the desired position in their mental ladders. They must position their brand to align with the patient's needs.

A brand positioning statement is a short written document describing how the marketer believes others should think, feel and relate to the brand. The brand positioning statement is about the customer. It is driven by the customer, identifying the target group's current needs and addressing those by offering compelling reasons to choose your brand. It is an internal document that acts as a roadmap for building the brand and realizing its full potential in the marketplace by compelling customers to choose it over the competition with its strategic communication.

Six Criteria

A brand positioning statement is not an advertising strategy, a slogan, or a tagline. Instead, it is a straightforward internal document communicated to all persons concerned to keep them aligned with the brand's objectives and aspirations. Therefore, you will find the following six criteria useful while creating your brand positioning statement.

1. **Relevance:** How relevant is our positioning to customers' needs? Do they care about it?
2. **Clarity**: Is our positioning clear enough for customers to understand?
3. **Credibility**: Is our positioning believable?
4. **Uniqueness:** Do our customers perceive our positioning as distinctly different from competitors' offerings?
5. **Attainability:** Can we deliver on what we promise in our positioning statement?

6. **Sustainability**: Is our positioning statement defendable? Is it difficult to imitate or copy by competitors? Can we maintain our distinctive position over time?

Superior Positioning Concept

Why develop a superior positioning concept? Because up to 90 percent of all new products fail, the figures may vary depending on the industry. For example, the new product success rate in the pharmaceutical industry is even lower, with only one in 10,000 molecules screened entering the market. The main reason for this high failure rate is that the core idea behind the product launch is not compelling and relevant enough.

Usually, most firms do not have a concept development process in place. However, some globally leading firms such as Proctor & Gamble, Unilever, General Mills, and Johnson & Johnson have been using the concept development process to design and develop new products for some time. The concept development process will help identify consumers' problems and their solutions in clear written statements and generate support and evidence that the solution can effectively address them. Lee Susen, Senior Director of New Business Development at E. J. Gallo Winery, suggests a six-step process to develop a superior positioning concept in his article, *Developing Superior Positioning Concept for A Product, Service, Idea or Experience*, published by the University of Virginia and Darden Business Press on September 5, 2018. These steps are:

1. Identify and prioritize new product opportunities
2. Identify consumer pain point(s)
3. Identify product/service to solve the consumer pain point(s)
4. Identify support and proof that your solution can effectively address the identified consumer pain point(s)
5. Test and validate the final concept
6. Integrate concept and product

After deciding and arriving at a superior positioning concept, it is time to position your brand precisely in the customer's mind so that he chooses your product. Lee Susen, in his above-mentioned article suggests four steps to position your brand successfully.

The Four Steps of Brand Positioning

1. *Define the context*: Since positioning is competition-oriented, you must understand the competitive scenario. What competitors do and customers think in the category you are competing in forms the context. It's all about what these customers think of your competitors, you and your company, and your brand.
2. *Find the differentiating idea*: A specialist differentiating idea is where a company does one thing differently or extremely well in a narrow or niche area. Hence, it does that *one* thing better than competitors that do more things. However, the specialist brand must stay focused on that one thing that it can do better than anyone else and not try to compete in other areas. The only limit of this specialist differentiated idea is that you cannot use it, if your market is too small as it will not be viable.
3. *Test the differentiating idea*: You need to test your differentiating idea, and there are two ways to do it— the *Opposite* and *Limits* test. **The Opposite test** asks whether anybody else has a brand positioning that is the opposite of yours. You have a problem if no competitor has an opposite brand positioning. Ask yourself who is saying the opposite of your differentiating idea. **The Limits test** is about finding the limits for your brand. Finding the *intrinsic* limits in your differentiating idea is useful because identifying and communicating your limits (a weakness) gives you a psychological advantage. Your customers will think you are honest and more open in what you say, even when you promote yourself.
4. *Brand positioning statement*: You need to remember three things when writing a brand positioning statement, which is an internal tool to manage your positioning.
    1. How can you remain focused on your brand positioning statement?
    2. How can you know if your message is right or wrong?

3. How can you teach your brand positioning to the whole company, new hires, suppliers, and partners?

Brand Positioning Statement (Template)

Four elements create the brand positioning statement, and these are:

- Target Patient
- The Brand Offering (Single-minded Proposition)
- Compelling Emotional Benefit
- Reasons to Believe

Typically, a brand positioning statement would be like this:

For (*target patient*), the brand provides (*single-minded proposition*) so that (*strongest emotional benefit*), because (*reasons to believe*).

Your brand positioning statement should follow two rules to be effective:

1. Your target audience (patients) should value the primary benefit in your strongest emotional benefit.
2. Your *Reasons to Believe* in your brand positioning statement should support your strongest emotional benefit.

The following table presents two examples of brand positioning statements.

Table 1.10 Brand Positioning Statement Examples

Brand Positioning Statements
Cialis
For couples suffering erectile dysfunction, *Cialis provides* a long-lasting effect allowing intimacy to happen spontaneously *so that* you can regain your relationship, *because* Cialis lasts for thirty-six hours.
Nexium
For GERD patients who are not getting better and are concerned about damage to their esophagus, *Nexium* provides fast relief and long-term so that you can feel better while protecting your stomach, *because* Nexium heals your esophagus lining.

Source: Markus Saba & Hilary Gentile, Brand Plan Rx: The Marketer's Guide to Building a Thriving health and Wellness Brand, BrightWing Media, 2021)

Assessing Your Positioning

How do you know your positioning is precise and aligned to address your patients' unmet needs and unaddressed pain points? It is accurate and precise if it meets the following criteria.

1. Is it *Unique* with a distinctive place in the category?
2. Is it *Believable* with irrefutable evidence to back our Promise?
3. Is it *Motivating* enough with a clear insight to activate the target customer?
4. Is it *Sustainable* and *difficult to imitate* and *copy* by the competition?
5. Is it *Single-minded* with a ruthless focus on one core reason for the customer to choose your brand?

Ground Rules for Positioning

Positioning is perception. Positioning is deciding what your product will do and for whom. The next step is making the customer perceive *it* the way you want him to. The key questions that one should ask and answer before positioning a product are:

a. What position do we already own in the prospect's mind? (for existing products)

b. What position do we want to own?

c. What is the *Gap* like?

d. What companies must be out-gunned if we are to establish that position?

e. Do we have enough marketing resources, both —money, and creative talent, to occupy the position we want to?

f. Do we have the conviction and guts to stick with the one consistent position?

g. Does our creative approach match our positioning strategy?

Let us now look at some ground rules for positioning a product. These are not rigid rules but some basic principles derived and formulated from a detailed and exhaustive study of several product successes and failures. Some important ground rules are:

1. **You cannot appeal to everyone:** There is no room for *panaceas* in the marketplace. A product that tries to appeal to everyone winds up appealing to no one. This attempt to appeal to everyone is, in fact, the antithesis of Positioning. If anyone claims that his product has a lot to offer, from *pediatrics to geriatrics*, in several conditions, a sort of *cure-all,* who will believe it? The credibility will be near zero, if not a real zero. Many pharmaceutical brands in India have achieved uncommon success through precise, non-ambiguous, no-nonsense Positioning.

   The following cases show how precise positioning helps brands to grow and, at the same time, how diluting one's position to appeal to more segments can hurt a brand.

CASE

20

Precise Positioning Improves the Blood Picture of Two Brands in the Hematinic Market!

Let us take the multi-hematinic market in India. It is a highly fragmented market with over a hundred plus brands. The market value was around Rs. 20 crores, with an annual growth rate of 1.2 percent in 1992. The majority of these brands do not have a clearly defined positioning strategy. A typical list of indications for a no-position hematinic looks like this:

In anemias due to diverse causes such as increased requirements of a hematinic during pregnancy, lactation, convalescence, malnutrition, restricted diet, obesity, chronic infectious diseases, tuberculosis, anorexia nervosa, chronic diarrhea, achlorhydria, post-gastrostomy, or gastro-jejunostomy, chronic hemorrhoids, hookworm infestations, etc.

Only two brands, Fefol of Eskaylabs (GlaxoSmithKline, now) and Livogen Capsules of Allenburys (GSK, now), had a clear positioning strategy. Both were positioned as *pregnancy haematinics*. Why? Because research indicated that pregnancy accounts for about 70 percent of hematinic usage. Fefol stayed with the theme *part of the routine of pregnancy and lactation* consistently.

They had put their might behind this position (the mother and baby contest was one unique promotional strategy they had adopted to reinforce their positioning strategy) and reaped a rich harvest of prescriptions.

Close on their heels was Livogen Capsules, which stayed with its strong, persuasive, and distinct theme, 11(blood-building factors) for the mother and 5 (mg of folic acid) for the fetus. This is not to say that the other hematinics were not promoted during pregnancy. On the contrary, pregnancy was one of the several indications in which other hematinic brands were promoted. In contrast, both Fefol and Livogen Capsules were positioned only in pregnancy and stayed in that position unwaveringly. Unflinchingly!

It has always been a neck-to-neck for Fefol and Livogen Capsules, with a negligible difference of less than one percent in terms of market share points, with Fefol having a market share of 11.6 percent and Livogen Capsules having 10.9 percent in 1992.

CASE

21

Clear Positioning Steers Glaxo Clear in Anti-Asthmatic Market!

Another case in point is Betnelan tablets of Glaxo (GSK, now). Each tablet of Betnelan contains 0.5 mg of betamethasone valerate, a potent corticosteroid, which can be used in many conditions like asthma, severe allergic disturbances, leukemia, rheumatoid arthritis, collagen diseases, various inflammatory skin diseases, nephrotic syndrome, ulcerative colitis, pemphigus, sarcoidosis (especially with hyper calcaemia), rheumatic endocarditis, ankylosing spondylitis, blood dyscrasias, agranulocytosis, and thromobocytopenic purpura, etc.

Betnelan, introduced sometime in the 1950s, was promoted in all these conditions till 1973. The company had a relook at its marketing strategies in 1973 and positioned Betnelan in bronchial asthma and promoted it vigorously. Betnelan achieved leadership and remained a strong leader for fifteen years after this clear, decisive Positioning in bronchial asthma. That is what clear, precise positioning can do to a brand.

The reason for this specific Positioning and its success with such a versatile drug like betamethasone valerate was that Glaxo was also marketing it in the same strength of 0.5 mg of the drug per tablet in a soluble tablet form under a different brand name, Betnesol effervescent tablets. Therefore, Betnesol tablets were positioned differently.

With its clear positioning strategy and the conviction with which it stayed, Glaxo achieved a formidable position in the systemic corticosteroid market, with a market share of 48 percent. Its positioning strategy paid off handsomely in marketing the twin brands of betamethasone very successfully. Both Betnelan and Betnesol continued to grow from strength to strength. There was no cannibalization of brands either. Positioning, clear Positioning had ensured harmony and growth instead.

CASE

22

Eli Lilly's Knee-Jerk Reaction to GlaxoSmithKline's Paxil Launch!

Eli Lilly, the global pharma major, launched Prozac (fluoxetine), the first SSRI (Selective Serotonin Reuptake Inhibitor) antidepressant, in January 1988. That became an unprecedented success and a blockbuster.

In 1992, GlaxoSmithKline launched Paxil (paroxetine), another SSRI agent, to treat depression.

Prozac was the market leader, and HCPs (Healthcare professionals) perceived it as more of an activating antidepressant useful for lethargic patients. However, GlaxoSmithKline positioned Paxil for depressed patients with anxious symptoms, a patient profile that matched its clinical benefits, and the company got FDA approval to treat SAD (Social Anxiety Disorder). Importantly, SAD (Social Anxiety Disorder) was a segment that was not yet developed., and therefore, no brand owned it.

Consequent to Paxil's launch, there was some decline in Prozac's market share. Seeing this, The Prozac team responded by moving away from its core positioning of an activating antidepressant to treat depressed patients with lethargy. Instead, it started highlighting Prozac's efficacy in relieving anxious symptoms associated with depression, trying to chase the new competition.

Prozac had a strong position in customers' minds as an effective antidepressant for the lethargic depressed patient as in stereotypical depression. However, as Prozac chased the competition, it was not only unable to change its position in customers' minds as an antidepressant that can relieve anxiety symptoms in depressed patients (Paxil's core positioning), but also started losing some of its base in its forte, which is *lethargic depressed patients*.

Prozac's new positioning confused customers, as it tried to be all things to all people, which is the antithesis of positioning. Prozac's loss of focus undermined its brand essence and eroded its market share.

Of course, Prozac course-corrected and got back to its core positioning—lethargic depressed patients, but its changing focus already damaged brand perception.

Prozac's knee-jerk reaction to competition eroded its market share and diluted its once formidable positioning in customers' minds.

(Source: Adapted from Source: Markus Saba & Hilary Gentile, Brand Plan Rx: The Marketer's Guide to Building a Thriving health and Wellness Brand, BrightWing Media, 2021)

2. **You Cannot Beat Them - The Brand Leaders Head On!**: Some positions cannot and should not be contested. For example, you cannot make a direct, frontal attack on the firmly entrenched brand leader. Over 2,400 years ago, Sun Tzu recognized the folly of attacking a superior and firmly entrenched competitor head-on. He said: *There are some roads not to be followed, some armies not to be attacked, some cities not to be seized, and some positions not to be contested.*

   If you wanted to introduce an antacid brand in the late 1980s, you would not be able to afford to attack either Gelusil or Digene. That would be setting you on a collision course. You could take a different position, but you should create differentiation and make your brand stand out. You should relate your product to the competition, but only to say that it is different and better than others. Your target audience must perceive it, and only then your differentiation would be meaningful.

   Unless your communication is based on a unique idea and position, the message is often put into the mental slot reserved for the leader in that product category. That is why with every addition of a new product that is not differentiated in a particular product group, the brand leader will gain share constantly, further strengthening its position. Here's a case in point showing how a new antacid made waves in the antacid, antiflatulent market.

CASE

23

The New Antacid's Guerrilla Warfare!

Biological E. Limited, in 1987 introduced a new antacid that jostled for space among a crowd of 151 antacid brands in a ₹ 450 million-large antacid, antiflatulent market. The company knew beforehand that it could not fight the brand leaders Digene of Boots (market share 19.9%) and Gelusil of Warner Hindusthan (market share 13.1%) head-on. Therefore, the company chose to create perceptible product differentiation. It formulated the product differently and promoted it as a *sodium-free antacid*. It caused enough dissonance since it has been common knowledge that sodium intake is restricted in hypertensive patients.

Furthermore, middle-aged patients who are susceptible to hypertension are also likely to be patients of hyperacidity. The company chose a different name for its brand that is suggestive and powerful enough to cut through the clutter. p*H4* is a highly suggestive name since that is the normal gastric pH level. The product became synonymous with normal gastric pH. The company reinforced its product differentiation in many ways and communicated persuasively about its differentiation. The net result is that the product found a *niche* for itself and gained a foothold in the minds of physicians, which no other antacid introduced during the previous six years was able to. While the new brand— pH4, did not take any share from the brand leaders, it certainly awakened the sleeping giants, who stepped up their promotional efforts to defend their market share.

(Boots later became a part of Abbott Healthcare and Warner Hindusthan, later became a part of Pfizer due to a series of acquisitions.)

3. **You Can Reposition Your Brand:** Even if you do not find any gaps in the market as it is currently defined and perceived, it may be possible to alter the market map and thus create new opportunities. For example, you can reposition your brand by introducing a new attribute and making it salient to the target market.

   It is a case of repositioning by changing the frames of reference, showing that you can reposition your brand against the competitor. Repositioning is undercutting an existing concept, or a product. One should not be afraid of conflict or controversy while repositioning a product. Consider these cases.

CASE

24

Alert makes it Good!

There are over a hundred antihistamines brands in India's anti-allergic market. Although many contain different ingredients, customers (doctors) continue to perceive these various brands as antihistamines with little or no difference. A few differences like *price,* which concern the dispensing or purchasing of doctors and hospitals, and *action of duration*, of course, existed in the served markets of different competitors. However, there were no major perceptible differences existed among the brands in the total market as such. It is because the brand leaders—Avil (Hoechst, Sanofi now) and Foristal (Ciba Geigy, Novartis) had been zealously guarding their respective served markets. All other brands had insignificant shares of the total market, with very few served markets.

Enter Incidal of Bayer. Incidal contained a different ingredient. Furthermore, with clear product differentiation and a clever repositioning strategy, Bayer invaded the served markets of various competitors and grabbed the business (prescriptions) right from under their noses. They promoted Incidal as an *Alert and Daytime Antihistamine* vigorously. It created a strong product differentiation in customers' minds as all other antihistamines cause drowsiness or sedation and cannot, therefore, be prescribed to patients while driving vehicles and who are busy at workplaces during the day. With its clear and clever repositioning as a *Daytime Antihistamine*, Incidal overcame the current limitations of all antihistamines in one stroke, stormed the antihistamine market, and achieved the second position in the market in a short span of a few years.

However, a few years ago, Incidal tablets are reformulated with cetirizine replacing the earlier active ingredient, mebhydrolin.

CASE

25

Repositioning Strategy Replaces an Entrenched Brand!

Here is an example of how Tylenol (a brand of acetaminophen) in the US was repositioned against the mighty Aspirin and won the battle. The Tylenol ads said:

For millions who cannot take Aspirin…if your stomach is easily upset, if you have an ulcer… or if you suffer from asthma, allergies, iron deficiency anemia, it will make good sense to check with your doctor before you take Aspirin… Aspirin can irritate stomach lining, and can cause hidden gastrointestinal bleeding… Fortunately, there is Tylenol…

Tylenol is a leading brand of analgesic antipyretic in the US, and many other countries. The repositioning strategy paid rich dividends indeed!

A few years later, an over-the-counter (OTC) brand of ibuprofen was trying to invade the served market of the mighty Tylenol brand with its repositioning strategy.

CASE

26

Synergistic Power of a Successful Repositioning Strategy!

Septran, the antibacterial that catapulted Burroughs Wellcome (GSK, now) into the limelight (from a mere ₹ 40 million company in 1973 to a ₹ 750 million giant in 1992), was repositioned against the mighty tetracyclines in 1973.

Septran was the Indian pharmaceutical industry's leading brand (sales ₹ 313 million, growth 3.1% in 1992). Septran, a combination of sulphamethoxazole and trimethoprim, positioned itself as an ideal alternative to the widely prescribed tetracyclines (rather indiscriminately used) that were reigning supreme up to the late 1970s. Particularly noteworthy is that the synergistic power of Septran, backed by the company's unprecedented promotional effort, pushed the brand to the dizzy heights of the industry's *number one* position even when other sulfa drugs were declining.

CASE

27

Late Entrant Emerges As A Leader in A Crowded Market Place!

In the late 1990s, antihypertensives were a crowded market in the United States pharmaceutical market. Novartis had launched its Diovan (Valsartan) as the second brand in the angiotensin II antagonists category. Merck's Cozaar (Losartan) pioneered the class two years before, in 1995. Close on the heels of Diovan's entry were two more significant competitors, Bristol Myers Squibb's Avapro (Irbesartan) and AstraZeneca's Atacand (Candesartan) in 1997 and 1998, making the market even more crowded. As a result, Diovan could only bank a disappointing $80 million in sales in its first year. Nevertheless, the brand team, Diovan, persuaded the top management to endorse a long-term strategy to establish the brand's presence.

The antihypertensive market in the US at the time was large and growing, with about 50 million hypertensive patients, including approximately 36 million untreated patients. The angiotensin II antagonists class was small, accounting for a mere eight percent of the market compared to the twenty-four percent for beta blockers and angiotensin-converting enzyme (ACE) inhibitors and twenty-one percent for calcium channel blockers (CCBs). The following table presents the details of their patent expiration:

Table 1.11 Patent Expiry Schedule of Diovan and Its Competing Brands

Brand	Patent Expires on
Norvasc (Amlodipine), the world's best selling antihypertensive	2007
Cozaar (Losartan) of Merck	2009
Avapro (Irbesartan) of Bristol Myers Squibb	2011
Atacand (Candesartan) of AstraZeneca	2011
Diovan (Valsartan) of Novartis	2012

The Diovan brand team started investing in a five-step relaunch strategy of Diovan following its disappointing launch performance:

1. Compete for out-of-class with angiotensin-converting enzyme (ACE) inhibitors and calcium channel blockers (CCBs) for first-line use
2. Differentiate from other angiotensin II antagonists in efficacy and selectivity
3. Pursue new indications, dosages, and combination products
4. Support all of the above with the most extensive clinical trial program in its class
5. Pursue an aggressive publication strategy in medical journals and increase the share of voice

The medical profession and the scientific community perceived the angiotensin II antagonists (AIIA) class as a second-line therapy at the time. Novartis' repositioning strategy of Diovan had helped the repositioning of the entire class of angiotensin receptor blockers (ARBs). However, Diovan had only a modest clinical advantage, the same efficacy as the leading ACE inhibitors and CCBs, and better tolerability. However, Novartis exploited Diovan's marginal advantage in its new global position - *Protective, Effective and Selective*.

Repositioning alone would not push Diovan's ranking in the marketplace. Cardiologists need clinical evidence, and Novartis did generate enough of it. So the company launched an aggressive Phase IV clinical program to support new indications and formulations. New indications included congestive heart failure, post-myocardial infarction, and high-risk hypertension, and obtained approvals from the FDA from 2002 to 2005.

Diovan's relaunch strategy did work effectively, and the brand team did deliver. As a result, Diovan became a blockbuster by 2001. By 2007, it was generating a whopping $5 billion in annual sales. In 2010, Diovan passed $6.1 billion in sales, making it the best-selling drug in Novartis' history!

(Source: Adapted from Francoise Simon and Philip Kotler's book, *Building GlobalBiobrands*, The Free Press 2003)

Positioning or repositioning strategies discussed here may look obvious and over-simplistic. The simplicity is deceptive. One can apply the principles of positioning strategy after thoroughly analyzing the various aspects like the current position of the brand, the desired position, and the existing gap between the two. One should not mimic another product's theme just because it is similar or falls into the same product category. Such a practice of imitative strategy could be disastrous. Consider this case.

CASE
28

MeToo Strategy Meets with a Disaster!

Imitation may be the best form of flattery. But, it could falter when overdone or without proper analysis in marketing.

Inspired by the success of Tylenol's classic repositioning strategy, Burroughs Wellcome (GSK, now) in India marketed their brand of acetaminophen, Ridake (manufactured by Litaka Laboratories). The company had chosen the OTC route. Large ads for Ridake appeared in leading newspapers. The copy was almost similar to the copy of the Tylenol ads when it was introduced in the US many years ago. However, there was strong objection to these ads as they were hyper-critical of the popular Aspirin. Comparative (or combative) advertisements were almost non-existent in India. The resistance to their advertising strategy was so high that the company had to withdraw these ads. The company finally got rid of the product that was supposed to rid the pain (hence the name Ridake)!

4. **There is Not Much Room Over There!:** The human mind can no doubt store and process an incredible lot of information (about 12 billion bits of information is the estimated capacity of the human brain, but scientists say that hardly 10 percent of it is used by an average individual. The brightest seem to be using about 15 percent). According to Harvard psychologist Dr. George A Miller, the average human mind cannot deal with more than seven items simultaneously in its working memory. Ask anyone to name all the brands he can remember in a given product category. For a high-interest category, chances are they will hardly get past seven—usually, it is much less.

   Your product has to occupy one of the seven positions to be remembered, recalled, and successful. If your product fails to occupy one of the seven *rungs* on the product ladder in the prospect's mind, it has no chance of survival. In any product category, the few top brands (usually 5 to 7) account for about 90 percent of the market. The Indian pharmaceutical industry is no exception to this.

   Moving up the ladder is difficult, particularly when the above brands are firmly entrenched and the gap is wider. A detailed analysis of the competing brands and their positions is crucial before one climbs the ladder.

   If you have a new product, it is often better to tell the prospect what the product is not rather than what it is. That is because the mind has no room for what is new and different unless it is related to the old and matches prior knowledge.

   The classic example is that the first-ever automobile was positioned as a *horseless carriage*. Among cough syrups for children in India, a *non-narcotic* brand was the leader in the 1990s. Patients prefer (and therefore, doctors, too) a *pain-free* injection. In the anti-inflammatory market, *non-steroidal* drugs are preferred. *Non-staining* ointments are highly acceptable among topical preparations as they have a cosmetic appeal. *Sodium-free* and *Sugar-free* preparations are sought after by many a health-conscious person.

5. **Credibility is the Foundation for Success!:** The foundation of a successful positioning strategy is its credibility. Whether

it is possible to tell the truth, the whole truth and nothing but the truth is beside the point. Unless the consuming public believes the message conveyed by the product promotion, the positioning game is lost.

Many claim that they are different in a highly competitive, over-crowded, me-too, rather me-me-too market like the pharmaceutical markets, which are increasingly genericized. But merely claiming one is different will not create a unique, distinctive position. At best, it will change the *me-too* market into a *me-different* or *me-me-different* market.

Only when the consumers perceive the *difference* will the product be successful. The *desired position* for the product in the minds of consumers can be created only when the product differentiation is genuine. Both in words and deeds.

Finally, what is axiomatic about the whole positioning business is this: honesty is the best policy for an effective, successful positioning strategy.

After discussing about positioning concepts, cases and how to position your brand effectively, it is important that we also understand some don'ts of positioning or how not to position our brands.

The Seven Deadly Sins of Positioning

1. *Positioning for the best of both worlds*: It would be best if you did not position your brand as offering the best of both worlds for the patient. For example, claiming that your brand offers maximum efficacy with minimum side effects and risks will not be credible as your customers won't believe it.
2. *Overpromising the benefits*: Never overpromise the benefits your brand can provide. For example, Do not ever claim that your brand gives your patients their lives back.
3. *Do not over-communicate* by saying that your brand does everything. For example, it is the most powerful, safe, effective, simple, convenient, and cost-effective solution.
4. *Do not ever claim that your brand is highly effective for all patient groups*. For example, it is safe and effective in treating patients from pediatrics to geriatrics.

5. *Beware of Competitive Myopia*. Do not define your competition too narrowly, taking only the competitors in your face whose challenge is direct and immediate. Instead, look out for less obvious challengers, who may not be on today's radar screen but could be real and prove dangerous if overlooked.
6. *Do Not Position Your Brand as a First-line or Second-line Treatment*. That is its place in therapy. Instead focus on what your brand stands for.
7. *Do Not say Things Like—Your* Brand is the first and only approved brand, or the only one you can rely on, or your first choice, etc. That is not positioning but genericizing your brand.

What Could be a better way to conclude this chapter on Brand Positioning in Pharma than with a summary of ten steps to a winning positioning formula?

Ten Steps to A Winning Positioning Strategy

Poorly differentiated or undifferentiated positioning can kill a brand without realizing its potential. Therefore, you must position your brands distinctively to make them stand out in the sea of sameness.

Charlene Prounis suggested ten steps to product positioning in the pharmaceutical industry in her insightful article, *10 Steps to Product Positioning*, published in MM+M on February 7, 2007. Here is the gist:

1. Gather insights from physicians and patients in your brand's therapeutic area by conducting interviews. Consider asking questions to understand how physicians treat diseases and what drives their prescribing decisions, treatment options, and unmet needs to position your brand effectively. Physicians are your best source as they constantly compare products, which is a critical part of their job.
2. Understand and assess the competition. The key questions to ask are:
   - How competitors' products are positioned?
   - Do their attributes support their positioning statements?

- What are their key claims?
- How are they handling their promotion?
- How do competitors' products address the needs of physicians? Patients?

3. Study thoroughly to understand the clinical attributes, features, and therapeutic class, including treatment guidelines, algorithms, and other elements that help achieve the therapeutic class of your product and competitors' products.
4. Involve your team in the brand's positioning strategy by conducting brainstorming sessions and internal positioning workshops with them.
5. Creating positioning statements that offer tangible and emotional benefits. Here are two examples of how some leading Pharmaceutical companies struck an emotional chord with their creative positioning strategies.
    - The brand team at Merck captured the essence of the condition, osteoporosis, on the underlying emotional issues, such as the constant threat of fractures faced by women with low bone density surrounding it with the positioning statement— Fosamax helps you gain independence.
    - Pfizer's marketing team developed a winning positioning statement for their brand, Aricept (donepezil), used for treating Alzheimer's disease. Aricept's positioning statement promised that patients with Alzheimer's disease could stay at home and avoid institutionalization to emphasize the drug's effectiveness of symptom control, allowing caretakers to reasonably manage their care at home.
6. Test your positioning concepts with physicians in one-on-one interviews online or in person and measure their responses. Understand how relevant, unique, or compelling the positioning statements are to the physicians you interview.
7. Use qualitative research methods, such as psychographic and ethnographic research among current and potential customers, to uncover emotional connections to your brand.

8. Refine your positioning options with the help of qualitative market research.
9. Getting buy-in from all internal stakeholders about the positioning statement you finalized is important. Then, you must convince the entire team that the positioning statement is the right one for making the brand successful.
10. After arriving at a viable positioning statement and convincing your team, you need to write a creative brief to convert the concept into a detailed tactical plan and implement it.

A clear, no-nonsense, unambiguous positioning strategy can build a sustainable brand in the highly competitive marketplace and even the company itself. There have been many instances where brands, with their effective positioning, catapulted their companies into the top league. Here is a case that illustrates how a highly successful brand built a company and pushed it into the top five of the industry league table.

CASE

29

Glaxo: The House That Zantac Built!

Glaxo Holdings is the house that Zantac built. In 1989, Zantac became the best-selling drug in the world, accounting for more than half of Glaxo's $4.4 billion in revenues. Zantac was launched in the United States in 1983, after its successful 1982 launch in Europe.

Glaxo Holdings PLC of Great Britain had a reputation as a somewhat conservative, if not stodgy, organization till the late 1970s. Then, however, its anti-ulcer drug, Zantac, a me-too new drug product that became the market leader, made Glaxo a global contender in the highly competitive pharmaceutical industry.

In 1983, when Zantac was launched in the United States, Glaxo was ranked sixteenth in the world pharmaceutical industry; by 1992, it became number two! During that period, Glaxo's market value grew four-fold, from $ 4 billion to 36 billion!

Zantac's exceptional sales contrast with its relatively ordinary medical performance. For all its achievements in the marketplace, Zantac was not a first-in-class drug. Instead, it was a me-too copy of SmithKline's pioneering antiulcerant drug Tagamet (Cimetidine).

In the late 1970s, Glaxo was effectively UK-based. The purchase of Meyer Laboratories Inc, in 1978, gave the company a foothold and an R&D base in the United States. Initially and until Zantac was launched, its sales from the US were relatively insignificant. In the first half of the 1980s, more than two-thirds of Glaxo's sales revenues were from Europe, Africa, and the Middle East. Zantac's launch in the US changed all that. The company moved into top gear and moved onto a new growth trajectory.

A Brief History of Anti-ulcer Drugs

One of the significant new products in the 1970s was the discovery of Cimetidine, the first histamine-2 receptor antagonist for treating ulcer disease. Cimetidine was discovered by James Black and his team of scientists at the British Laboratories of SmithKline & French (GlaxoSmithKline now). Cimetidine was launched as Tagamet late in 1976 at a Royal College of Physicians symposium. By 1981, Tagamet was achieving nearly $ 300 million in sales in the United States.

In the late 1970s, Glaxo's scientists also worked on histamine-2 receptor antagonists, which are analogs of Cimetidine (Tagamet). The anti-ulcer market, thanks to Tagamet, was growing rapidly. So Glaxo scientists worked on improving Cimetidine by overcoming its limitations and side effects. Glaxo, in the process, discovered Ranitidine, which it named Zantac.

Launched in 1981 in the United Kingdom and Italy, Zantac had the following advantages over Tagamet:

1. Zantac needed to be taken twice a day, whereas Tagamet had to be taken four times a day.
2. Zantac had fewer side effects as compared to Tagamet.

Glaxo had made great use of its advantages over Tagamet in its promotional campaigns in copybook style. Zantac's phenomenal success had catapulted Glaxo from a medium-sized British pharmaceutical company into the top ranks of the world pharmaceutical industry. To the enviable Second position by 1989.

Glaxo mounted a classic two-stage operation in textbook style to get Zantac into the huge and lucrative US market. In the first phase, between 1983 and 1989, Glaxo forged a co-promotion strategy with the Swiss Pharma Major, Hoffman-La Roche. In the second phase, from 1990 to 1994, Glaxo rapidly consolidated the success of Zantac by building its marketing workforce in the United States to sell what was an established product.

Key Elements of Zantac's Strategy

Glaxo decided to market Zantac not as a Tagamet monopoly breaker but as a major evolutionary advance in treating peptic ulcers and other acid peptic disorders. This was rather unusual for a second product in the drug class. This was a major strategic decision that guided all others in Zantac's winning game plan.

Paul Girolami, Glaxo's Chairman and Managing director himself, assumed the responsibility of developing the launch marketing plan for Zantac. He began with a focus on the physicians' needs. He knew that an anti-ulcer drug's ability to relieve the patients' pain and heal the ulcer (healing rate) were the two prime characteristics that influenced the physicians' selection of anti-ulcer therapy.

Questioning Tagamet's safety was a neat line of attack. It was Glaxo's very aggressive positioning strategy to attack its rival, where it is more vulnerable. This is particularly so when Glaxo could not prove that Zantac was better. It had not been used widely enough for its side-effect profile to emerge. But by the same logic, it could not be disproved. Glaxo made skillful use of this information and conveyed it as a decisive advantage to all key stakeholders, such as physicians, patients, and payors. Although Tagamet had proven its safety in trials and over time in use, it had certain side effects such as nausea, diarrhea, drowsiness, decreased sperm count, gynecomastia, and drug-drug interactions. These side effects of Tagamet had proved to be Zantac's window of opportunity. And Glaxo turned Tagamet's weaknesses into Zantac's strengths, using aggressive advertising to give information-hungry gastrointestinal physicians the evidence they needed to prescribe Zantac.

Girolami and his marketing team decided to alleviate selected side effects through product refinement and then attack Tagamet on those side effects. Tagamet could not deny them. Zantac, as a result of product refinement, did not have them. So Zantac launched an aggressive marketing program highlighting its product superiority.

Glaxo had priced its second-in-class drug, Zantac, at a 20 percent premium over its rival, the first-in-class drug and market leader Tagamet. This, too, was unheard of in the industry.

Co-marketing of Zantac with the Swiss Drug Major Hoffman-La Roche in the United States was another master stroke in Zantac's strategy. Co-marketing alliances were necessary to get to the critical mass of appropriate sales levels for Zantac since Glaxo had a relatively small field force at the time of Zantac's launch. Roche, at the time, had an under-utilized sales force with the patents of its commercially successful products, Valium and Librium, running out. With this, more than 1,200 detail men started promoting Zantac's superiority to all gastroenterologists and PCPs across the country, rapidly increasing prescriptions and sales. Under the co-marketing agreement, Roche would detail and sell Zantac under the Glaxo brand name. Glaxo would pay Roche 40 percent of sales revenue for five years.

Glaxo had also used co-marketing strategies in France with Formin and in Germany with Cascina. Co-marketing helped the company reach the critical mass needed for Zantac in terms of sales volumes and market share.

Continuous and accelerated product development was another important element in Zantac's strategy. Zantac was an outcome of product development. Glaxo tweaked the Tagamet molecule, improved its side-effect profile considerably, and extended its action of duration. It also used parallel processing to cut the developmental time in half. Glaxo did not stop after discovering Ranitidine with these perceptible and patentable therapeutic advantages. It continued its development. When Tagamet responded to Zantac's attack on its dosing frequency with its twice-daily dosage version, Zantac continued to improve its dosing frequency to once daily. Zantac seized the product development initiative from its rival, Tagamet. Further, Glaxo continued with many line extensions for Zantac in terms of different strengths, dosage forms such as liquid, pediatric dosage forms such as Baby Zantac, and injectables. The pioneer, Tagamet, responded to most of these but a bit late.

The GERD indication approval for Zantac in 1986 was probably one of the most important features of its strategy. It offered Zantac a major advantage. Glaxo created GERD, which grouped many symptoms related to gastrointestinal disorders such as heartburn, acid reflux, etc., and called it Gastro Esophageal Reflux Disorder. Before the FDA approved treating GERD with Zantac, heartburn... did not seem to warrant a prescription drug. It was perceived to be well managed by over-the-counter remedies. Glaxo had elevated the medical importance of GERD condition by presenting it as an acutely chronic *disorder* with an underlying physiologic etiology and the potential for serious longer-term consequences if left untreated.

Glaxo created an Institute for Digestive Health, which sponsored its research and equated GERD with more serious gastrointestinal diseases simply by discussing it in the same context. One of the institute's missions is to raise public awareness about issues relating to digestive health. The branding of GERD not only shifted the public perception of the dangers of chronic acid reflux but also put Zantac in the spotlight as the best overall solution. It also implied that acid blockade rather than acid neutralization is necessary as it attacks the root of the condition before it manifests itself and does the damage.

The GERD indication approval enlarged the market considerably. Because GERD is a condition that occurs more commonly and in a relatively larger population, it is also treated by primary care physicians more often and not just by gastroenterologists. In addition, Zantac was the only product that received FDA approval to treat GERD for quite some time. Tagamet got approval for the treatment of GERD almost five years later, in 1991. As a result, GERD accounted for almost two-thirds of Glaxo's annual $ 2 billion sales of Zantac.

Last but not least, overcoming the traditional marketing mindset was also a key factor in Zantac's success. Pharmaceutical companies at the time used to think of themselves as highly specialized, hanging in on their target markets of doctors and hospitals, pharmacists, and wholesalers as if they were packaged goods consumers. However, when it came to marketing Zantac, the company thought differently. Zantac's marketing strategy evolved from close studies of the marketing tactics of some of the leading consumer goods success stories, such as McDonald's, Nutrasweet, and Perrier.

Glaxo used a very wide range of marketing techniques across multiple channels to promote Zantac. For example, the company has conducted several educational symposia, issued numerous consumer awareness bulletins, public service announcements via radio and television, Journal advertisements, etc. Glaxo also introduced many formulations of Zantac for different age groups and medical practice settings and extended many therapies for long-term maintenance. All these initiatives gained a larger market share for the company and successfully expanded the market for anti-ulcer drugs.

Racing for the Anti-ulcer Market

The anti-ulcer drug market as we know it today started in 1977 with the introduction of SmithKline & French's Tagamet in the United States. Until the entry of Zantac in 1983, SmithKline did not have to bother about competing for market share in the histamine-2 receptor antagonist market as it had one hundred percent of the market to itself under its patent status. Tagamet's marketing goal was to convince more physicians of its therapeutic benefits and improve the rate of adoption of its new therapy.

When Glaxo introduced Zantac in 1983, the monopoly of Tagamet had become a duopoly. There was an additional marketing goal. Tagamet had to preserve its market share against Zantac among those doctors who were currently prescribing Tagamet. Zantac detailers, too, had a twin objective before them. They had to convince the doctors who had not yet taken up the new therapy to take up Zantac for treating their patients with duodenal ulcers and take a share from the current prescribers of Tagamet by convincing them about Zantac's superiority over Tagamet and consequent therapeutic benefits to their patients. Thus the marketing rivalry had begun in the anti-ulcer drug market between Tagamet and Zantac.

Two more competitors in the histamine 2 receptor antagonist market, Pepcid of Merck and Axid of Eli Lilly, entered in October 1986 and April 1988, respectively. The competitive noise had increased. So did the market expansion, with more players drumming up their versions of the H2 receptor antagonist story in treating acid peptic disorders. In 1989, a new class of drugs for treating GERD and ulcers, Prilosec (Omeprazole, discovered by Astra of Sweden and marketed by Merck in the USA), was also approved by the FDA, further intensifying competition. The following table presents important milestones of the race for the anti-ulcer drug market.

Table 1.12 Racing for the Anti-ulcer Drug Market: Key Milestones

Timeline	Event or Activity
August 1977	US FDA approves Smithkline's Tagamet (Cimetidine) for the short-term treatment of duodenal ulcer
April 1980	US FDA approves Tagamet for the long-term maintenance treatment of duodenal ulcer
December 1980	US FDA approves Tagamet for the treatment of gastric ulcer
July 1983	US FDA approves Glaxo's Zantac (Ranitidine) for the treatment of duodenal ulcer
July 1984	Glaxo's Zantac captures 25 per cent of Tagamet-Zantac market within one year of its launch
May 1986	US FDA approves Zantac for the treatment of GERD (Gastro Esophageal Reflux Disorder) an indication created by Glaxo

Table 1.12 *Contd...*

Timeline	Event or Activity
October 1986	US FDA approves Merck's Pepcid (Famotidine) another histamine-2 receptor antagonist for the treatment of duodenal ulcer
January 1988	Zantac overtakes Tagamet in total sales
April 1988	US FDA approves Eli Lilly's Axid (Nizatidine)
September 1989	US FDA approves Merck's Prilosec (Omeprazole discovered by Astra, Sweden and marketed by Merck in the United States) a first-in-class proton pump inhibitor drug for the treatment of GERD
March 1991	A. US FDA approves Tagamet for the treatment of GERD B. Zantac becomes the first-ever drug in the world to reach $ 1 billion in sales
June 1991	US FDA approves Prilosec for the short-term treatment of duodenal ulcer
May 1993	The market shares of the four histamine 2 receptor antagonists were: Zantac 55 per cent; Tagamet 21 per cent: Pepcid 15 per cent; Axid 9 per cent
1994	Zantac becomes the best selling drug in the world with almost $ 4 billion in annual sales

Zantac continued to race past its competitors in the anti-ulcer drug market. Zantac was truly prodigious in its performance right from its birth throughout its life cycle. It had many firsts to its credit. The first-ever prescription drug crossed the $1 billion mark in global sales. Also, it was the first-ever prescription drug to cross the $4 billion mark in global sales.

Speaking about Zantac's phenomenal success, Martin Preuveneers, Director for International Marketing, remarked in 1992: *The sales of Zantac were very close to those of Jaguar and just a little more profitable.*

Lessons

The anti-ulcer drug Zantac is a classic study of a successful, late-entering product. Zantac was superior to the pioneer anti-ulcer drug, Tagamet, in important ways:

1. it had fewer side effects
2. It had a more convenient dosage schedule, twice-daily as compared to the four-times daily of Tagamet

By waiting and entering later, late movers can cash in on the pioneer's efforts in creating the market and outmuscle them. Late movers can also tweak their products to convert the pioneer's weaknesses into strengths. Besides this almost axiomatic principle, Zantac offers many more lessons for pharmaceutical marketers. Consider these, for example:

1. Top management commitment is crucial to establish a new brand. Paul Girolami, the Chairman and Managing Director of Glaxo at the time, had led the development of Zantac from strategy to execution. Even in India, when Glaxo launched Zantac as Zinetec, the involvement of Humayun Dhanarajgir, the managing director of Glaxo, India, in the launch strategy and subsequent management of the brand was unprecedented.
2. Attack the competitor where he is most vulnerable. Make the competitors' weaknesses your strengths, wherever they are relevant to patient benefits.
3. Once you tweak your product and make it better than your major competitors, do not rest on your laurels. Think of improving your product continuously. To make it more useful to the patients. Listen to their needs. Understand and respond.

4. Marketing is about differentiation. Think differently, and study the success stories of other industries. Apply the lessons where relevant.

(Source: Adapted from article—Paul Rodgers, The House that Zantac Built: Glaxo Pins its Hopes on A New High-tech Research Center in Stevenage, Independent, February 5, 1995)

CHAPTER

2

Disease Branding

Disease Branding is about seeing old diseases in new ways.

— Vince Parry, Brand Strategist, and Author of the book, *Identity Crisis: Healthcare Branding's Hidden Problems and Proven Strategies to Solve Them*

Disease Branding

Disease branding or branding of a condition has been gaining importance in pharmaceutical marketing for some time now. Pharmaceutical marketers and healthcare practitioners are taking it to a new level of sophistication. Branding a condition is gaining prominence as it helps the Pharma brand managers and clinicians stay focused on the same theme and structure of the problem, and solution surrounding a disease condition. In other words, it keeps them both on the same page.

Origins of Disease Branding

When did the branding of a condition or disease begin? How did the pharmaceutical industry get the idea of branding a disease? You can get the answers to these questions and understand where the Pharma industry got the idea of branding disease from a 1928 book, *Propaganda*, by Edward Bernays. Many consider Bernays as the father of public relations in America. Carl Elliot narrates the interesting case that throws light on the origin of disease branding in his book, *White Coat, and Black Hat*.

How do you brand a disease or condition? It is pretty straightforward. First, you need to define a particular condition and its associated symptoms in the minds of physicians and patients. Second, you must predicate and offer the best treatment for that condition.

The concept of branding a disease condition is by no means new. The first-ever disease branding effort dates back to the 1920s when Warner and Lambert (Pfizer now) successfully branded a condition—Halitosis. However, the landscape for branding a disease has become more complicated today. It includes pharmaceutical companies, external thought leaders, support groups, and patient communities. The success of branding a condition depends on how you can build consensus among the diverse groups that matter internally and externally. When done appropriately, the disease branding follows the structure of a lock and key story, where the lock is the problem or the disease, and the key is your product, which is a solution for the problem condition.

Dual Advantages

Branding a disease offers significant benefits to the company both internally and externally. Internally, the activity rallies the entire team's support by motivating them and creating a sense of ownership among all the members. The product, too, can better own the customer perceptions about current and evolving disease states and define new patient segments. The product can also reinforce its position by meeting unmet needs and providing greater therapeutic benefits.

Externally, the branding effort of a company-sponsored activity helps forge better relationships with the thought leaders. At the same time, they are engaged in debating and shaping the new therapeutic approaches with the physician community. As a result of all this significant initiative and effort, the brand creates a leadership status as the owner and driver in the new category.

Three Strategic Approaches

How do you brand a disease or condition? Three principal strategies help you create a disease condition and align it with your product:

1. Elevating the importance of an existing condition
2. Redefining a current condition to reduce a stigma
3. Developing a new condition to build recognition for an unmet need.

Five Questions

Vince Parry, president and chief branding officer at Parry Branding Group, a leading Pharma branding consultancy company, suggests five questions to find out whether disease branding is right for you in his article, *The art of branding a condition* published in Medical Marketing & Media on May 1, 2003.

1. Does your product uniquely impact a disease condition? Does it work via a new pathway or at a new site of action? Does it address an underlying cause, attack the root of the problem, or relieve symptoms that would benefit from redefining (branding) the disease to highlight the difference?
2. Are there any stigmas or social concerns about the condition your product treats that would hinder a physician-patient dialogue?

3. Does your product significantly benefit a condition with little or no awareness?
4. Are there competitive efforts to reposition your product as beneficial in only a niche condition that is not perceived as an essential health risk?
5. Are you seeking a niche within a crowded therapeutic category?

Benefits of Disease Branding

Detractors criticize disease branding as empty profiteering. However, the truth is that disease branding does provide certain benefits. Consider these, for example:

- New understanding of diseases that have been around for many years
- Awareness of little-known conditions
- A more positive (or less negative perception) of a disease
- Seeing old diseases in new ways
- Removing frustration and confusion about certain old disease conditions by understanding the underlying pathology and new approaches to treat them
- New understanding leads to more awareness and cognizance of seriousness and legitimacy.
- Eliminating stigmas surrounding certain disease conditions

To brand a disease is to shape its public perception to make it more palatable to potential patients. Not very long ago, people regarded many conditions such as bad breath, panic disorder, reflux disease, erectile dysfunction, bipolar disorder, overactive bladder, attention deficit hyperactivity disorder (ADHD), premenstrual dysphoric disorder (PMDD), restless legs syndrome (RLS) and many others as rare, until a marketing campaign transformed the trend.

Here are some classic cases where disease branding has been successfully used.

CASE

30

Pharma's first shot at disease branding!

Warner Lambert's Listerine offers a classic example of a solution looking for a problem. Humans had bad breath from time immemorial. Ancient peoples had spent centuries searching for a cure for bad breath. Finally, a pharmaceutical company created a medical condition out of bad breath, offered treatment, and made huge profits.

Warner and Lambert invented Listerine in the 1880s. Listerine was named after Dr. Joseph Lister (1817-1912), who was the father of modern antiseptics. Listerine was originally marketed for various conditions such as dandruff, foot cleaning, and even floor cleaning. Later, people used to apply it to wounds or areas that were likely to be infected. They used it as a surgical antiseptic, not a mouthwash like we do today. The company later found that Listerine would work very well in killing germs in the mouth. The company also moved Listerine from a prescription-only-medicine (POM) to over-the-counter (OTC) status. Although the sales gradually increased, that was not enough for the founder, Jordan Wheat Lambert. He wanted more. Finally, his son came up with a brilliant idea. He found a new name for bad breath— Halitosis. The company adopted the word from the Latin word, 'Halitus,' which means bad breath. The word 'Osis' makes it sound more medical. The new name for bad breath made people with bad breath believe that they had a treatable condition. Unfortunately, bad breath had a stigma surrounding it. People were shy to speak about it and were even avoiding social contact. Friends and relatives who noticed it also would keep quiet and maintain a safe distance. Also, bad breath had negative consequences ranging from social casualties, such as lack of career advancement, to divorce. Nobody believed that bad breath could be treated. Warner-Lambert changed it all by creating awareness — and anxiety — and a severe-sounding medical condition, Halitosis.

The new name for bad breath, Halitosis, quickly transformed the social stigma and gave confidence to people that they could treat it with Listerine. They felt confident marching into the drug stores and nowhere else since the advertisements stressed that, "Your closest friends won't tell you about the problem" and asking for the cure. The creative advertising for Listerine not only increased the awareness of the condition among the public but also made Listerine a household name.

Listerine ran many advertisements in many newspapers and magazines talking about the sad unmarried Edna, who remained single as she watched her friends getting married. It's not that she wasn't a great gal! It's just that she had this condition (bad breath)! Here is one of the most successful and memorable ads of Listerine with a very persuasive copy:

Often a bridesmaid...Never a bride!

Most of the girls of her set were married...but not Eleanor.

It was beginning to look, too, as if she never would be.

True, men were attracted to her, but their interest quickly turned into indifference.

Poor Girl! She had not the remotest idea why people dropped her so quickly... and even her best friends wouldn't tell her.

No Toothpaste Kills Germs

Like Listerine... Instantly.

Listerine antiseptic does for you what no toothpaste does.

Listerine instantly kills germs by millions. Stops bad breath (Halitosis) instantly, and usually for hours on end.

Far and away is the most common cause of bad breath is germs.

You see, germs cause the fermentation of proteins, which are always present in the mouth.

And research shows that your breath stays sweeter longer the more you reduce germs in the mouth.

Toothpaste with the aid of a toothbrush is an effective method of oral hygiene. But, no toothpaste gives you the proven Listerine Antiseptic Method – banishing *bad breath with super-efficient germ-killing action.*

Listerine Antiseptic Chemically Proved Four Times Better Than Toothpaste

Is it any wonder Listerine antiseptic in recent clinical tests averaged at least four times more effective in stopping bad breath odors than the chlorophyll products or toothpastes it was tested against? Every night… before every date, make it a habit to use

Listerine is the most widely used antiseptic in the world.

Listerine Antiseptic Stops Bad Breath

4 Times Better Than Any Toothpaste

Many companies today medicalize problems and brand disease conditions to solve them. However, Listerine was medicalization's first and most famous success story!

(Source: Brainiac, How Claude Hopkins Manipulated the World to Use Toothpaste—Pepsodent Hopkin's History, kickstartersidehustle.com)

CASE

31

The Mother of all Disease Awareness Campaigns!

You develop and market a new drug that meets the unmet need. That is a simple, straightforward view of drug development and marketing, as we know. Sometimes, the drug development and marketing process as we know and understand it may be entirely different. Picture this, for example. First, pharmaceutical company scientists develop a drug with various physiological effects, none of which are very helpful. Then, marketers are driven to identify and promote a disease for the drug to treat, which is drug development in reverse order. It might mean co-opting a relatively rare illness and thinking of ways to expand its borders to increase the prospective patient pool.

Merck's promotion of amitriptyline (Elavil) in the 1960s offers a classic example of this strategy. Amitriptyline was a new antidepressant useful in the treatment of clinical depression. However, in the 1960s, clinical depression was regarded as a rare condition offering minimal scope in marketing it profitably as an antidepressant.

The solution is rather obvious. Increase the frequency of diagnosis. Expand the patient pool. Merck came up with the idea that set a trend of increasing disease awareness. The mother of all disease awareness campaigns that were to follow later. What did Merck exactly do? Merck bought fifty-thousand copies of a book by Frank Ayd called, *Recognizing the Depressed Patient* and sent them free of charge to general practitioners all over the country. Prescriptions for Elavil (amitriptyline) increased dramatically following this strategic attempt to increase the frequency of diagnoses even though another antidepressant, imipramine, has been available since the mid-1950s in the market.

The sales of antidepressants were never depressing since then. On the contrary, from a few million dollars in the 1960s, the market for treating depression has grown to multi-billion dollars in the next thirty years.

The key to selling antidepressants became clear: to sell clinical depression.

(Source: Adapted from Carl Elliott's book, White Coat, Black Hat)

CASE

32

The Birth of A New Condition - GERD!

In 1986, When Glaxo (GlaxoSmithKline now) launched Zantac for ulcers, it faced the challenge of broadening its reach into the heartburn market. Heartburn, at the time, did not seem to warrant treatment, not certainly a prescription drug. The heartburn sufferers were managing their condition with many available over-the-counter remedies.

To enter the large heartburn segment by expanding the usage of its Zantac, Glaxo had to elevate the medical importance of heartburn to an acutely chronic disorder with an underlying physiological etiology and the potential for severe longer-term consequences if one does not treat it. The company launched a well-coordinated initiative to achieve this. The term heartburn, coined decades ago by antacid brands suggested that the mechanism of action in the treatment of indigestion is acid neutralization, which is what antacids do. However, research in the 1980s suggested that chronic heartburn could further be described as a malfunction of the esophageal sphincter. This more serious disorder can lead to the erosion of gastrointestinal tissue over time.

Glaxo and Zantac worked to rebrand chronic heartburn as a more serious medical concern that you cannot afford to ignore. Glaxo coined a new term for heartburn and many other associated symptoms and grouped them into one condition, Gastro-Esophageal

Reflux Disorder (GERD), thus giving heartburn the status of a medical condition, warranting treatment. Through this rebranding of the condition, Glaxo could put Zantac in the spotlight as the best overall solution. It suggested that you should stop the problem at its root, which is the blockade of acid, and not at its symptom level, which neutralizes the acid.

Glaxo created the *Glaxo Institute of Digestive Health (GIDH),* a platform for education and awareness of digestive diseases. The GIDH sponsored research awards in gastrointestinal health and discussed Gastrointestinal Esophageal Reflux Disorder (GERD) in the context of other, more serious gastrointestinal (GI) diseases. In addition, the company engaged with powerful third-party advocates such as the American College of Gastroenterology (ACG) and fielded a massive public relations effort called *Heartburn Across America*.

The result? Glaxo doubled the number of physicians who were leaders in gastrointestinal (GI) health, which helped the company drive the annual sales of Zantac to a whopping US $2 billion. What is even more interesting about this is that about two-thirds of this revenue is from prescriptions for GERD!

(Source: Adapted from the article—Paul Rodgers, The House that Zantac Built: Glaxo Pins its Hopes on a New High-tech Research Center in Stevenage, February 5, 1995, Independent)

CASE

33

Upjohn's Efforts in Disentangling Panic Disorders from Anxiety Disorders Pay Handsome Dividends!

The development of Xanax in the 1970s and the creation of Panic Disorder in DSM III (Diagnostic and Statistical Manual for Mental Disorders III Edition) offer an excellent example of the condition-branding strategy.

In anxiety and depression, as the illness is rarely based on measurable physical symptoms, they are open to conceptual definitions. Over the years, the increasing number of identified emotional conditions has resulted from breaking the problems into different conditions to better access treatment options. Pharmaceutical companies funded the research and publicity of many of these newly coined disease conditions.

In the Diagnostic and Statistical Manual of Mental Disorders - II (DSM-II), panic disorder fell into the broad category of anxiety neurosis. Patients experiencing panic attacks, as there was no clear branding of the condition at the time, often visited cardiologists thinking their problem was a heart condition. Cardiologists, too, labeled those complaints as cardiac complaints and the patients hypochondriacs due to a lack of physical pathology.

Dr. David Sheehan, a pioneering thought leader in panic disorders, helped characterize the conditions and push for a new way to diagnose and treat them. Upjohn, the maker of Xanax (alprazolam), helped fund this early research. His research helped characterize panic disorder and paved the way to diagnose and treat it. Furthermore, Upjohn had given an unrestricted grant to the National Institutes of Mental Health (NIMH) to organize a three-day thought leader conference that resulted in a published consensus on the diagnostic criteria for panic disorder and how best to treat it. As a result, in 1980, the DSM-III listed panic disorders as a new diagnostic category.

Upjohn had a clear strategy for developing alprazolam (Xanax) in the 1970s. According to Dr. David Sheehan, the company's strategy was to take advantage of the medical profession's confusion in classifying anxiety disorders. The company wanted to create a perception that the drug (Xanax) had special and unique properties that would help capture market share and displace Diazepam from the top position. There was, in fact, nothing unique in this regard about Xanax. Benzodiazepines were all good for panic disorder. However, only Upjohn got the US FDA approval for its Xanax in treating panic disorder in doses up to 6 mg daily (equivalent to 20 to 120 mg of Diazepam).

Xanax was the first to receive panic disorder as an exclusive indication, thereby maintaining its leadership position in anxiety disorders. Upjohn aggressively marketed its Xanax in panic disorders. In addition, the company has published research articles in all the relevant scientific journals and arranged speaking tours for cardiologists to raise their awareness of the heart-brain connection in the minds of panic-disorder patients. It is perhaps no coincidence that panic disorders have grown over 1,000-fold since the 1980s!

(Source: Adapted from Vince Parry's article on *Branding a condition*, Medical Marketing & Media, May 2003)

CASE

34

Pfizer Eliminates the Stigma Surrounding Impotence with an Acronym!

Some conditions are medically relevant, with considerable social stigma and embarrassment surrounding them. The stigma surrounding these conditions is often worsened by many over-the-counter (OTC) remedies, whose low-brow promotional efforts push patients further into hiding. Male impotence is one of those conditions. It has long existed as a medical condition. Still, even the medical profession in the past associated it with disability linked to physical trauma or, more often, a loss of libido. The patriarchal society always looked down upon the persons with this condition as inadequate, contributing to the low self-esteem of the sufferers. Even the remedies over the years were often invasive, and their implementation indiscreet.

Pfizer redefined this embarrassing medical condition by renaming it as erectile dysfunction (ED) and eliminating its stigma. Furthermore, with its brilliant and hugely successful effort of linking the newly named condition with its new drug, Viagra (sildenafil citrate), Pfizer showed the millions of patients who have male impotence that it is treatable. The term erectile dysfunction (ED) changed the focus of the condition from being associated with lack of potency or male virility to the more enlightened concept of a reversible physical loss of function. Like other recognizable conditions such as GERD (Gastro Esophageal Reflux Disease), and OAB (Over Active Bladder), the company captured the condition of male impotence in an acronym—

ED. ED makes it suitable for direct-to-consumer promotion and functions as an easy password between physician and patient to initiate a formerly difficult conversation. ED gave a kind of empowerment to its sufferers.

The simple, discreet, and empowering brand personality of ED has met its match Viagra, which is an elegant and effective solution for this redefined condition.

(Source: Adapted from Vince Parry's article on *Branding a condition*, Medical Marketing & Media, May 2003)

CASE

35

Eli Lilly Fields A Second Brand of the Same Drug for A Branded Condition!

The Diagnostic and Statistical Manual for Mental Disorders (DSM) first mentioned Premenstrual Dysphoric Disorder (PMDD) in 1987. The 1993 edition, DSM IV, repackaged and renamed the condition giving it a new life. PMDD is a severe form of premenstrual syndrome (PMS).

In June 1999, with the patent of Prozac about to expire, Eli Lilly organized a roundtable discussion inviting the PMDD subcommittee members to build a consensus regarding the diagnosis and treatment of PMDD and to get approval for Prozac. Approval for Prozac for treating PMDD would give a seven-year extension for Prozac. To get approval, Lilly needs to establish that PMDD is a real condition and Prozac is the right treatment.

Shortly after the roundtable discussion, an article, "*Is premenstrual dysphoric disorder a distinct clinical entity?*" appeared in the Journal of Women's Health and Gender-Based Medicine and emerged as the state of the science. It was the outcome of the roundtable discussion. The authors, probably recalling their description of earlier research (before DSM IV) as sparse and poor, claimed that later evidence proved PMDD to be a real condition and Prozac to be an effective treatment. However, only a few articles were post-DSM IV Research and did not provide substantial evidence that post-menstrual mental illness exists. Most of the articles constituted the promotion of Prozac by reporting that Prozac improves symptoms of women with the premenstrual dysphoric disorder (PMDD).

The FDA's Psychopharmacological Drugs Advisory Committee (PDAC) met on November 3, 1999. Eli Lilly representatives brought PMDD Subcommittee member Jean Endicott, the first author of the roundtable article, to speak. At the end of the meeting, there was a consensus among the PDAC members that PMDD is a clinical entity that is well defined and has accepted the diagnostic criteria.

In July 2000, the US FDA granted Interneuron Pharmaceuticals Inc., based in Lexington, Massachusetts, the approval for Sarafem (fluoxetine) in treating premenstrual dysphoric disorder (PMDD). Lilly received the US and global patent application rights for marketing Sarafem under an agreement with Interneuron Pharmaceuticals. Sarafem is the first and only prescription medication indicated for PMDD. Eli Lilly sponsored a pre-launch activity to build awareness for the new condition, recasting diagnosis to conform to the new criteria. The result was a fascinating integration of PMDD awareness and Sarafem brand strategy.

Lilly decided on a dual brand strategy for its fluoxetine— Prozac for depression and Sarafem for PMDD. The additional brand— Sarafem, will give it a distinct identity, which will help with its educational efforts for the mostly under-recognized condition, PMDD. It would also reduce confusion about the differences between depression and PMDD. Prozac is primarily associated with depression, and women with PMDD are not depressed. So Lilly needed a new name to effectively distinguish the new patient group (potential PMDD sufferers) from Prozac's association with depression.

Lilly's marketing team did create a distinct personality for their new brand of fluoxetine for treating PMDD. It started first the name itself— Sarafem. 'Sarafem' in Hebrew means 'Angel,' a word with female overtones befitting the target patient group. Its packaging, too, amplified the female associations. The Sarafem tablet came in a pretty pink-and-lavender shell. The company created a wonder cure aura around the brand for this distinctly female condition – premenstrual dysphoric disorder.

Eli Lilly followed a multichannel marketing strategy to promote Sarafem. Its advertising messages flooded the airwaves immediately after the FDA approved Sarafem to treat PMDD. The following advertisement illustrates the kind of advertising effort the company had put: The ad shows a woman who has lost her keys and is increasingly frustrated. The voiceover breaks through:

Think it's PMS? It could be PMDD - premenstrual dysphoric disorder. You know these intense moods and physical symptoms the week before your period. Sound familiar? Call for free information about PMDD and your doctor's treatment to relieve its symptoms. Why put up with this another month?

In addition to its direct-to-consumer advertising, Lilly had launched a marketing campaign targeting psychiatrists, gynecologists, and mental health providers and sent them promotional materials such as flyers, free samples, invitations to Lilly Talks, and visits by their pharmaceutical representatives. The massive promotional effort spread the word around the medical community, quickly increasing the diagnoses of PMDD. When the diagnoses soar, can sales be far behind? They, too, soared.

(Source: Adapted from an article by Caplan, Paula J, Premenstrual mental illness: *The truth about Sarafem (premenstrual dysphoric disorder and the usage of Sarafem (Prozac) as treatment*, The Network News, May 2001)

CASE

36

Positioning A Brand by Creating A Disease!

What would you do if you had a drug that relieves some of the annoying symptoms of a disorder that is not very common, and patients do not seek even treatment because they are embarrassed to share their condition? Drop the drug and move on to the next drug candidate in the development phase. Many marketers might do that. Drop the drug from marketing because it is unviable, but not Neil Wolf, the group vice president of Pharmacia (now Pfizer). He was different and thought differently, and spotted a tremendous opportunity. Here is what he did with a little-known disorder and the drug to treat it.

Pharmacia found that its new drug, tolterodine (Detrol), was useful in treating urge incontinence. However, there was just one major problem. The market for incontinence in the United States was very small — about $40 million, with generic Oxybutynin having annual sales of $29 million. Also, the disease prevalence was very low, around 5 to 15 percent, mainly affecting elderly patients 65 years and above. When it came to the pharmacotherapy of the condition, only about a fifth of the patients in this small segment of the patient population were treated with prescription drugs. Therefore, it was a significantly under-diagnosed and under-treated condition.

What is the solution? Neil Wolf, the group vice president who later steered the global launch of Detrol, came up with a brilliant strategy.

Broaden, and expand the market. More importantly, understanding the market in all possible dimensions, such as clinical, epidemiological, psychometric, and economic, created a commercial opportunity that was attractive enough. Pharmacia had to convert a niche product into a mass market opportunity. The company had to:

1. Increase the diagnosis and treatment of incontinence
2. Expand the appropriate patient population beyond urge incontinence

To increase the diagnosis and treatment of incontinence, raise awareness of the disease — urge incontinence, which is not currently perceived as a disease as it was thought to be a consequence of aging. Change that perception and make the patients and physicians understand that urge incontinence was a disorder and treatable with medications. In other words, created a disease in the minds of the patients and physicians that urge incontinence was a treatable disorder. And then position Detrol as the treatment for that disorder. More importantly, change the name and definition of urge incontinence to Overactive Bladder.

Why change the name? The overactive bladder is highly intuitive and marketing-oriented compared to the earlier names — incontinence or detrusor instability. Detrusor is a muscle that controls the process of storing and releasing urine by its contraction and relaxation. The name — overactive bladder — immediately suggests a picture of something you can recognize and associate with. In addition, experts say that the name change helped in making the condition more acceptable for public discussion. The patients were able to bring it up with their doctors without embarrassment. Meanwhile, those doctors were encouraged to screen patients for this condition and to keep them on their medication once it was diagnosed.

Creating and increasing awareness about the condition of the overactive bladder among physicians was the next significant step that Pharmacia took. As early as 1996, Pharmacia identified two major key opinion leaders, Alan Wein of the University of Pennsylvania and Paul Abrams of the University of Bristol in England, for its new drug under development, tolterodine (Detrol), which is found to be useful in the treatment of incontinence. These two well-known KOLs held their first conference on the overactive bladder in London in June 1997. As a result, Wein And Abrams became known as the godfathers of an *overactive bladder* disorder. Pharmacia, which had been doing pioneering work on overactive bladder drugs, sponsored the conference.

Pharmacia's public relations work, too, had been exemplary. In December 1997, six months after the first conference on overactive bladder, the leading journal of the Urology field — *Urology*, published a special supplement on the overactive bladder with about thirty articles on the condition. In addition, Wein and Abrams wrote the introduction in which they talked about a promising new drug, Detrol, manufactured by Pharmacia.

The US FDA approved Detrol on March 25, 1998. By 1999, the International Continence Society (ICS) was writing a new definition of overactive bladder, which expanded the number of people who met the diagnostic criteria. Pharmacia's groundwork in illness inflation was beginning to pay off. Drug companies drive disease inflation to create or expand the definition of conditions that are part of everyday life and to create treatment guidelines for drugs designed for those conditions.

In 2001, Pharmacia sponsored the National Phone Survey, which asked a variety of questions about the urinary habits of Americans. The survey asked 5,204 adults questions about how often they needed to urinate, whether they had to get up at night and whether they felt the urgency.

The company wanted the condition — of overactive bladder not only to be recognized by both patients and primary care physicians but also to create an environment where they own the condition.

Pharmacia got what it wanted from this survey. The results produced a striking number: Nearly 17 percent of adults in the United States — about 33 million people were deemed to have overactive bladder disorder. So a massive new market for Detrol was born.

Pharmacia, through its significant efforts at KOL-level, Phase IV research activity, and active participation at the first ICS (International Continence Society), was able to change the earlier name of the disorder of overactive detrusor to the overactive bladder at the Overactive Bladder Consensus Conference in July 1999. The new definition is: *OAB (overactive bladder) is a medical condition referring to the symptoms of frequency and urgency, with or without urge incontinence when appearing in the absence of local pathological or metabolic factors that would account for these symptoms*.

Accordingly, Detrol tablets are useful for treating urinary frequency, urgency, or urge incontinence symptoms. A case of the disease that is tailor-made for the capabilities of the drug!

Now that the indication had been defined as it was intended, the next logical step in Pharmacia's game plan was to create an environment where primary care providers perceive overactive bladder as a serious condition and not a consequence of aging. Also, to make it easy to screen, diagnose and treat OAB. Later, in January 1999, the company followed it up with a DTC campaign in print media to increase screening and diagnostic rates. The copy of the print ads was somewhat like this:

If you think you have an overactive bladder... Let your doctor know how symptoms affect your life...Your doctor needs to know more about your symptoms. He or she should also know how it affects your life. If you recognize even one of these signs, fill out the questionnaire and discuss it with your doctor:

1. Do you go to the bathroom so often at night that it interrupts your sleep two or more times?
2. Do you go to the bathroom so often that it interferes with the things you do (usually more than eight times in 24 hours)

3. Do you always have to know where the bathroom is because of frequent, strong sudden urges to urinate?
4. Do you sometimes not make it to the bathroom in time?
5. Do you wear pads to protect your clothes from wetting?

These are some of the typical signs of an overactive bladder. Occasionally, some may be associated with other more severe conditions. If you have any of these symptoms, contact your doctor.

Pharmacia established overactive bladder as a serious condition and not just a consequence of aging among patients and physicians but also all other key stakeholders, such as payers and regulators. Last but not least, the company established superiority over oxybutynin, the existing treatment option for urge incontinence. As a result of this marketing blitz, Pharmacia achieved greater than 90 percent unrestricted access to Detrol among managed-care lives.

Table 2.1 Time Line for Detrol Positioning and Creating the Overactive Bladder Condition.

Timeline	Activity
1996	Pharmacia begins its activity to develop and engage key opinion leaders to educate physicians and patients about its new drug under development, Detrol (tolterodine), which is useful in the treatment of incontinence.
1997	Alan Wein of the university of Pennsylvania and Paul Abrams of the University of Bristol in England hold their first *Overactive Bladder* conference in June. Pharmacia sponsored the conference.
1997	Urology, the leading medical journal of the field publishes a special supplement on *Overactive Bladder* with about thirty articles on the condition in the month of December.
1998	US FDA approves Detrol.
1999	International Incontinence Society expands number of people who meet the criteria with its new definition of Overactive Bladder
2001	Pharmacia sponsors a National Phone Survey among 5,204 adults asking a variety of questions about urinary habits of Americans.
2002	Neil Wolf, group vice president, who was in charge of global launch of Detrol makes a slide presentation on how the company tried to promote their new drug.

With a well-thought-out, creatively crafted strategy, Pharmacia made a little-known, under-diagnosed, and under-treated niche-condition like urge incontinence into a mass-market opportunity by converting it into the overactive bladder. The following table presents a snapshot of the company's achievements with Detrol in less than five years.

Table 2.2 Detrol's Marketing Success

Marketing Criteria	1997	2001
New Prescriptions	1.5 million	4.6 million
Treated Patients	3.6 million	12.7 million
Detrol Sales	-	400 million
Detrol Prescriptions (Market Share - %)	-	50.2

How did Detrol achieve such remarkable success with an insufficient, insignificant opportunity? By broadening disease definition and simplifying screening and diagnosis, Pharmacia expanded the patient population and differentiated Detrol from Oxybutynin.

In sum, Pharmacia created a disease (Over Active Bladder) out of almost nowhere (urge incontinence, which was thought to be a consequence of aging, and not a disorder) and positioned its new drug, Detrol, to treat the new disorder, OAB!

(Source: Adapted from Neil Wolf's (Group President, Pharmacia) powerpoint presentation on Positioning Detrol (Creating A Disease) to PMRG (Pharmaceutical Marketing Research Group) on October 7, 2002)

CASE

37

A Disorder Made to Order!

SmithKline Beecham (Glaxo SmithKline, now) received approval for its Paxil (paroxetine hydrochloride) from the US FDA in May 1996 for the treatment of panic disorder and obsessive-compulsive disorder (OCD). The company was lagging in the antidepressant market, where Pfizer's Zoloft was the market leader. SmithKline wanted to bridge the gap and move rapidly in the market. The company was in search of a new indication that would help it grow quickly.

Glaxo SmithKline hired Cohn & Wolfe, a public relations firm specializing in the pharmaceutical industry, well-known for its unconventional ways of marketing. The company wanted Cohn & Wolfe to lay the groundwork for the introduction of Paxil. They identified a new condition, social anxiety disorder (SAD), under-diagnosed and under-treated at the time. Diagnostic and Statistical Manual of Mental Disorders IV (DSM IV) listed Social anxiety disorder for the first time, replacing the earlier term — generalized social phobia. DSM IV defined social anxiety disorder as "*marked and persistent fear of one, or more social or performance situations in which the person is exposed to unfamiliar people or possible scrutiny by others.*"

The task before SmithKline and Cohn & Wolfe, their public relations firm, became clear. The company obtained approval from the US FDA for Paxil in treating social anxiety disorders in 1999. Once the company got its approval of Paxil for SAD, SmithKline turned its attention to the task of promoting the disease itself. To promote social anxiety disorder as a severe condition. They had to convince shy people that they suffer from social anxiety disorder and need treatment. They formulated and followed advertising and public relations blitz campaigns with multiple activities. Consider these, for example:

1. By early 1999, the PR firm created a slogan, *"Imagine being allergic to people,"* and wallpapered bus shelters nationwide with pictures of a SAD-looking man vacantly playing with a teacup. The copy read: *You blush, sweat, shake — even find it hard to breathe. That's what Social Anxiety Disorder feels like.* The posters did not refer to Paxil or SmithKline. Because if you make any reference to the brand or the company that makes it, you need to mention all the risk factors and side effects. Therefore, the posters bore the insignia of the *Social Anxiety Disorder Coalition* and its three non-profit members, the *American Psychiatric Association (APA)*, The *Anxiety Disorders Association of America,* and the *Freedom from a Fear* advocacy organization.
2. The coalition was not a grassroots alliance of patients suffering from anxiety disorders or other mental illnesses. SmithKline assembled it quickly, and its PR firm, Cohn & Wolfe, handled all the media inquiries on behalf of the group.
3. Cohn & Wolfe did not stop with posters. The firm also created a video news release, a radio news release, and a Matte (a bylined article that smaller newspapers often run unedited) release. The PR agency gave a press packet that stated: *SAD affects 13.3 percent of the population or 1 in 8 Americans and is the third most common psychiatric disorder in the United States after depression and alcoholism*. However, this information contrasts with what the DSM sites. According to DSM, studies show that between 3 and 13 percent of people may suffer the disease at some point in their lives, but only 2 percent experience enough impairment or distress to warrant treatment.

4. A few months after the FDA approval of Paxil for SAD, SmithKline launched a series of advertisements touting its efficacy in helping patients with social anxiety disorders in braving dinner party situations and public speaking occasions.
5. SmithKline also had psychiatrists as paid consultants for conducting SAD trials for Paxil and making TV appearances.
6. Cohn & Wolfe, the PR agency, also supplied journalists with expressive patients to put a face on the disorder. PR firms handpick patients, give them media training and send them on promotional tours to help publicize a disease condition.
7. GlaxoSmithKline also recruited celebrities like Ricky Williams, the NFL (National Football League) running back, to give interviews to the press about their social anxiety disorder.
8. Also, the company hired academic psychiatrists working on social anxiety disorder and sent them out on the lecture circuit in the top 25 media markets.

The results of the company's massive advertising and public relations thrust were remarkable. In the two years before SmithKline received the FDA approval for Paxil, there were hardly fifty references to social anxiety disorder in the popular press. However, in May 1999, when the FDA approved Paxil for social anxiety disorder, hundreds of stories about the condition— SAD appeared in the US publications such as the New York Times, Vogue, Good Morning America, and several television news programs.

By 2001, Paxil had become the seventh most profitable brand in America. In addition, Cohn & Wolfe had picked up an award for the best PR campaign of 1999. In less than two years, GlaxoSmithKline took a once-considered-rare psychiatric condition and helped it transform into a major epidemic called social anxiety disorder, claiming that 1 in 8 Americans suffer from it. This transformation pushed Paxil's sales to the US $3 billion a year in the process!

(Source: Adapted from Article: Brendan L. Koerner, Disorders made to order, Mother Jones, July/August issue 2002)

CASE

38

Two Stories: How ADHD Was Sold, and How Two Brands Dominated the ADHD Market!

Attention Deficit Hyperactivity Disorder (ADHD) was virtually unknown in 1956, when the Swiss Pharma major, CIBA-Geigy, started marketing Ritalin (methylphenidate), the most widely used drug for ADHD today.

It was only in 1980 that the American Psychiatric Association (APA), in their publication of the third edition of the Diagnostic and Statistical Manual of Mental Disorders (DSM-III), included Attention Deficit Disorder (ADD) for the first time, including the subtypes— ADD with hyperactivity and ADD without hyperactivity, and ADD residual type.

Attention deficit disorder (ADD) — the condition for which Ritalin (methylphenidate) is most commonly prescribed was formerly called hyperactivity, as reflected in its alternative acronym: Attention Deficit Hyperactivity Disorder (ADHD). Its diagnosis is based on problems with Attention, focus, impulsivity, or overactivity at school or home.

In 1990, ten years after the condition was first mentioned in the DSM III, about 900,000 children and adults were diagnosed with ADHD. And less than a decade later, the number of diagnoses swelled to five million. The growth of this magnitude in ADHD diagnoses suggested a problem of epidemic proportions.

The sharp rise in ADHD diagnosis was directly tied to another startling statistic — a 700 percent increase in the amount of Ritalin (methylphenidate) produced during the same period. An increase in this proportion was unprecedented and alarming for a single drug, particularly when it was considered a controlled substance.

In later years, the sales of stimulant medications for treating ADHD have soared from about $1.7 billion in 2002 to a whopping $9 billion in 2012, according to IMS Health.

ADHD: A Historical Timeline

How did the number of diagnoses and the sales of ADHD medications show such phenomenal growth? What factors contributed to this? Before we explore further the causes and reasons behind this enormous growth, let us quickly take a quick look into the historical timeline of ADHD and how it came to be what it is now. ADHD-brain.com presents the timeline of ADHD history:

- In 1902, Sir Frederick Still, the well-known English pediatrician, first described children with symptoms like ADHD and thought that the children with these symptoms had a defect of moral control.
- In 1908, Alfred F. Tredgold, an influential writer and medical expert in the early decades of the twentieth century in Great Britain, described high-grade feeble-minded children who likely had a form of mild brain damage that caused them to have ADHD-like anti-school behavior.
- In 1937, Dr. Charles Bradley, a Rhode Island physician, discovered that using benzedrine in children with behavior problems improved performance in a residential and school setting. Investigations from his work later led directly to the current pharmaceutical treatment of ADHD.
- The year 1952 marked the publication of the first edition of the Diagnostic and Statistical Manual of Mental Disorders by the American Psychiatric Association (APA). It does not mention ADHD-like disorder.
- In 1957, hyperkinetic impulse disorder was used to describe for the first time to describe children with ADHD symptoms.

- Herbert Freed and Charles A Pfifer studied the use of Thorazine (chlorpromazine) on hyperkinetic, emotionally disturbed children in 1957.
- In 1963, Dr. Carmen Keith Conners, an American psychologist best known for establishing the first standards for the diagnosis of attention deficit hyperactivity disorder (ADHD), published a study on the effects of Ritalin (methylphenidate) in emotionally disturbed children.
- In 1966, minimal brain dysfunction syndrome became a popular term for children with various combinations of impairment in perception, conceptualization, language, memory, and control of Attention, impulse, or motor function.
- In 1967 and 1968, the National Institutes of Mental Health (NIH) gave researchers many grants to study stimulants' effectiveness on children with ADHD symptoms.
- In 1968, the American Psychiatric Association (APA) published the second edition of the Diagnostic and Statistical Manual of Mental Disorders (DSM-II). It included the disorders — hyperkinetic reaction of childhood or adolescence, and organic brain syndrome.
- In 1969, Dr. Keith Conners published the first Conner's Rating Scale, which eventually led to revised editions of the Conner's Rating Scales for parents and teachers.
- The Washington Post published a story describing how 5 to 10 percent of all school children in Omaha and Nebraska were receiving stimulants like Ritalin to control their behavior, even though the statistics in the story were a subset of students who were in specialized programs. However, the story seemed to imply that 5 to 10 percent of all students in Omaha were on stimulants. Also implied in the article was that many parents were being coerced to put their children on a stimulant. This fueled a major controversy around the overuse of medications in students and the over-diagnosis of ADHD.
- In 1970 and 1971, the Comprehensive Drug Abuse Prevention and Control Act created a separate class for drugs with the

highest potential for abuse and addiction. As a result, stimulants such as methylphenidate were added to the Schedule II class, placing tight controls on their prescribing and refills.

- The Rehabilitation Act of 1973 added ADHD as a qualification for additional help and services at school for children with ADHD to help them succeed.
- In 1975, the anti-Ritalin movement gained momentum. Several books were published to reinforce the belief that ADHD is not a real diagnosis and hyperactivity is caused by food allergies and additives and is not inherited. Further, it was a condition created by drug companies to make more profits.
- In 1980, The Association for Academic Psychiatry (AAP) published the first statement about ADHD and Medication for hyperkinetic children, which says that in addition to consideration of non-drug therapy situations where such an approach is appropriate, there is a place for stimulant drugs in the treatment of hyperkinetic children.
- Also, in 1980, the American Psychiatric Association (APA) published the third edition of the Diagnostic and Statistical Manual of Mental Disorders (DSM-III), which included, for the first time, Attention Deficit Disorder (ADD), including the subtypes— of ADD with hyperactivity, ADD without hyperactivity, and ADD residual type.
- In 1981, Dr. Russel A Barkley, professor of clinical psychiatry at the medical university of South Carolina, USA, wrote the first of 17 books about ADHD— *Hyperactive Children: A Handbook of Diagnosis and Treatment.*
- In 1987, APA published the DSM-III-R. This edition changes the name of ADD to ADHD but does not name subtypes.
- Also, in 1987, the American Academy of Pediatrics published a special report: *Medication for the treatment of children with Attention Deficit Disorder* containing guidelines and indications for drug therapy in its treatment ,naming several stimulant drugs and tricyclic antidepressants as being potentially useful.

- In 1993, Dr. Russel A Barkley started publishing, *The ADHD Report Newsletter*.
- In 1995, Dr. Joseph Biederman published one of the first hundreds of medical studies about children with ADHD.
- In 1996, AAP published an updated report: *Medication for children with attention disorders*, which stressed that drug therapy should be combined with appropriate management of a child's environment and curriculum.
- In 1999, NIMH (National Institutes of Mental Health) published results from a 14-month study known as the Multimodal Treatment of ADHD study (MTA Study); it involved 570 children with ADHD at six sites in the United States and Canada. It showed that medication alone was more effective than psychosocial treatments alone, but their combination was more beneficial.
- In 2000, APA published DSM-IV-TR naming three types of ADHD - including ADHD combined type, ADHD inattentive type, and ADHD predominantly hyperactive/impulsive type.
- Also, in 2000, the AAP published its clinical practice guidelines, including diagnosing and evaluating children with ADHD and giving clear clinical guidelines for pediatricians and parents on assessing and treating children with ADHD.

Adults: The New Frontier of ADHD

Undoubtedly, the children's market for ADHD has been very profitable for the drug industry. However, it is still limited. However, a much larger market for adult ADHD is looming. But how should a doctor diagnose adult ADHD? First, Eli Lilly, the maker of Concerta (methylphenidate), sponsored the efforts of some academic ADHD specialists at Harvard and New York University to create a diagnostic ADHD questionnaire that could be used in adults. Later, the World Health Organization (WHO) endorsed a slimmed-down version of the questionnaire. Big Pharma then spent considerably on public awareness campaigns about the illness. Consider these highly influential campaigns narrated by Alan Schwarz in his book *ADHD Nation,* for example:

- Dr. Ned Hallowell, ADHD guru and child psychiatrist, on an episode of ABC's The Revolution in 2012, along with the show host, Ty Pennington, performed a quick ADHD exam on an adult audience member. After the test, he concluded: *So you passed the test. Welcome to the illustrious club (of ADHD). It's a good news diagnosis... there is a medication that people are afraid of but should not be. The medication works about 80 percent of the time. And when it works, it works like eyeglasses! ...You can suddenly see!*
- Later, Dr. Hallowell, with the same level of enthusiasm that goes beyond the evidence, said in an interview with Gwyneth Paltrow's lifestyle website, GOOP: *If you are an adult reading this, and you feel you are underachieving, learn more about ADHD. It could be the answer you've been looking for years. Diagnosis and treatment would replace frustration and underachievement with success. The diagnosis of ADHD and the treatment that follows, if done properly, truly can change a life, at any age, from frustration and underachievement to one of triumph, fulfillment, and joy.*

Can you think about promoting the diagnosis and treatment of serious mental illness by promising a solution to all life's problems? Of course, that is how you effectively sell a product.

Globalization of ADHD

ADHD diagnoses and prescriptions skyrocketed in the US. However, the trend of increasing diagnoses and prescriptions for ADHD in other parts of the world has been growing significantly, if not to the same extent as in the US. For example, between 2007 and 2012, methylphenidate prescriptions increased by 50 percent in the United Kingdom. In 2013, the global consumption of methylphenidate increased to 2.4 billion doses, a 66 percent increase from the year before. The United States, however, accounts for more than 80 percent of global consumption.

Peter Conrad, and Meredith R. Bergey, medical sociologists, both, vehemently criticize the medicalization of ADHD in their paper on *the impending globalization of ADHD: Notes on the expansive growth of a medicalized disorder* in Social Science & Medicine, in December 2014. Here is the gist of what they said in their article:

- The principal concern of the authors is that ADHD is being medicalized. Children of different age groups who may be merely naughty or high-high-spirited are being misdiagnosed with ADHD, and are wrongly treated with powerful medications such as Ritalin.
- Five major causes are driving the global expansion of ADHD and its subsequent medicalization: drug industry lobbying, the influence of US-based psychiatry; the adoption of user criteria for diagnosis; the influence of ADHD patient advocacy groups; the growth of information on the internet.
- In the past, drugs for ADHD were heavily marketed in the US, which is getting saturated. The drug companies, therefore, are looking for greener pastures and expanding into the international markets to promote their ADHD medications aggressively. The markets they have been targeting are—Western Europe, Japan, Mexico, and Brazil, among others.

That is how ADHD, a medical condition requiring treatment with stimulants and non-stimulants, has evolved into a multi-billion dollar market. The ADHD market is expected to experience significant growth in seven markets, such as the US, France, Germany, Italy, Spain, the UK, and Japan, to reach $13.9 billion by 2024, according to Global Data, a research and consulting firm. Two brands have mainly contributed to the phenomenal growth of the condition and the market. They are Ritalin of Ciba-Geigy (Novartis now), the Swiss drug major, and Adderall of Shire Pharmaceuticals, a leading global biotech company with Dublin, Ireland, as its headquarters.

Big Pharma Sponsors Biederman Studies

Dr. Joseph Biederman, unequivocally the most published psychopharmacology maven for ADHD, had conducted many clinical studies on the effectiveness of psycho-stimulant drugs in treating attention disorders. Pharmaceutical companies sponsored most of these studies. The findings of these studies gave credibility to the treatment of ADHD with stimulant drugs by giving three essential messages:

1. The disorder was under-diagnosed.
2. Stimulants were effective and safe.
3. Unmedicated ADHD led to significant risks for academic failure, drug dependence, car accidents, and brushes with the law.

Ritalin and Adderall, through their brilliant marketing efforts, first marketed ADHD as a condition and then offered their brands as a solution to treat the problem of ADHD. Ritalin started it all, and Adderall reinforced it with all its might and had been reaping rich rewards from the ADHD market. Therefore, the story of Ritalin and Adderall marketing is also the story of marketing ADHD. Ritalin first!

How Ritalin (methylphenidate) Marketed ADHD?

Before we go into the details of how Ritalin rode the market with ADHD, an interesting tidbit about how Ritalin got its name. Leandro Panizzon, a chemist at Ciba (Novartis, now), synthesized methylphenidate in the early 1950s. He shared his invention with his wife, Rita, who tried the medication on herself. To the couple's delight, Rita enjoyed tennis, and methylphenidate had an excellent effect on her tennis game. So Leandro named the new drug in honor of his wife. He named the new drug Ritalin.

Ciba began marketing Ritalin in 1956, in the United States for a wide range of adult psychiatric disorders. However, evidence was emerging that it might improve the behavior of disturbed children, as they were then called. In 1963, child psychiatrist Leon Eisenberg and child psychologist Carmen Keith Conners, who was then working at the Johns Hopkins Hospital, published a landmark article based on their clinical studies that showed methylphenidate improves children's behavioral symptoms. The diagnostic label, attention deficit hyperactivity disorder, did not exist yet. However, the article, *The effects of methylphenidate on symptomatology and learning in disturbed children* by Eisenberg and Conners in The American Journal of Psychiatry in November 1963 put the drug on the child psychiatry map.

Journalist Alan Schwarz, in his hard-hitting book, *ADHD Nation: Children, Big Pharma and the Making of an Epidemic*, narrated an episode that explains how the involvement of Ritalin and, indeed, Big Pharma began in selling ADHD, following the famous methylphenidate clinical trial by Eisenberg and Keith Conners. Here's the story:

Some weeks after the publication of Conner's and Eisenberg's paper in the American Journal of Psychiatry, the authors, received a man in a suit, who showed up at Eisenberg's office. The visitor gratefully glided a slip of paper across his desk as Conners looked on, saying, "For further studies." But unfortunately, the visitor was a representative from Ciba, and the note was a check for $5,000. Eisenberg tucked the check into a desk drawer, warned Conners to "watch out for these guys," and never spoke of the day after that.

That's how the long and enduring engagement of Ritalin in the marketing of ADHD began. Since that $5,000 check from Ciba, Schwarz says that pharmaceutical money has irrigated the channels running through every corner of the ADHD ecosystem, feeding researchers, patient advocacy groups, celebrity spokespeople, and advertisers.

In the late 1960s, when direct-to-consumer advertising was not allowed in the US, Ciba found a smart way to persuade parents to test and treat their children for ADHD. They distributed pamphlets to parents through the teachers in the schools their children were studying. Ciba representatives in that district provided these pamphlets to the schools. The pamphlet contained a logo of the company Ciba on the backside. One of such brochures read: *Parents should be aware that these medicines (stimulants such as methylphenidate) do not drug or alter the child's brain. Instead, they make the child normal.*

Targeting the Teachers

Targeting doctors, nurses, and patients is a normal and established practice for pharmaceutical companies. Pharma companies had started targeting teachers for marketing their ADHD medications even before direct-to-consumer advertising was approved in the US. As teachers have some concerns and play an important intermediary role in diagnosing and treating ADHD, pharmaceutical companies have designed many ways to reach and influence them. For example, Novartis, the manufacturer of Ritalin, created an educational website with specific content for teachers. On one page entitled *If Parents Ask*, for example, Novartis suggests responses teachers might make to concerned parents:

Make it clear to them that it is important for them — and their child — to understand and follow the doctor's medical advice about medication and other therapies for ADHD. ADHD is a serious condition that may require the child to be on medication and undergo counseling for a longer duration.

Further, the site incorporates links to the company, or directly to Ritalin (medication produced by the manufacturer) for a discussion on the diagnostic process and references to the legislation regarding access to medication. Another pharmaceutical company, Shire Pharmaceuticals (manufacturer of Adderall), has an annual toll-free *Ask The Experts ADHD hotline*. Experts provided for this hotline include teachers, school nurses, doctors, and advocates. The suggested topics include the management of ADHD in school.

Furthermore, in 1997, Novartis collaborated with the National Association of School Nurses in the US to run a nationwide campaign, providing 11,000 school nurses with a resource kit containing information on ADHD and its treatment and various support organizations. In addition, the company extended the collaboration to produce a resource to curb the misuse of psycho-stimulant medication providing links to Novartis Pharmaceuticals.

Sixty-plus and Still Counting...

It has been sixty-four years since Ritalin was launched, and the drug continues to have a significant presence in the treatment of ADHD. Even though there have been many competitors since its patent expired, eroding its sales and profits, the importance of methylphenidate is very much present. Notable among the competitors is Adderall, which Shire Pharmaceuticals markets. It is Adderall that took the mantle and eventually the leadership position in expanding the ADHD market when Ritalin lost its market exclusivity. Here's a timeline of methylphenidate that reinforces its continued importance in ADHD treatment.

Methylphenidate (Ritalin) Timeline

1955 Ritalin (Novartis)

1982 Ritalin SR (Novartis)

1999 Metadate ER (methylphenidate extended-release - Cell Tech Pharmaceuticals)

2000 Methylin ER (Methylphenidate extended-release - Novartis)

2000 Concerta (Methylphenidate - Janssen Pharmaceuticals)

2001 Metadate CD (Cell Tech Pharmaceuticals)

2002 Ritalin LA (Novartis)

2005 Focalin XR (dexmethylphenidate - Novartis incensed from Celgene)

2006 Daytrana (methylphenidate patch - Noven Pharmaceuticals)

2012 Quillivalant XR (Liquid Methylphenidate - Next Wave Pharmaceuticals)

2016 QuilliChew (Methylphenidate chewable tablets - Pfizer)

Adderall, the New Leader

The loss of exclusivity of Ritalin opened the doors of fortune for the company to invent a new drug to treat ADHD, get approved and patented, then unleash it on the awaiting market. Schwarz notes that *this is par for the course for big Pharma: when a patent dies, a new brand drug must rise — even if the new one is not one iota better*. Enter Adderall. How it entered the market and later conquered is a curious and interesting story.

The story of Adderall starts with a decades-old weight loss drug called Obetrol. The US FDA withdrew its approval for this drug as early as 1973. However, Rear, a small pharmaceutical company, kept selling it for weight loss until the 1990s without approval. Rear was not selling much Obetrol, but interestingly a pediatrician in Utah was writing an unusually high number of drug prescriptions. He was using it for ADHD.

Around the same time, Roger Griggs, a high school football coach, started a small pharmaceutical company named Richwood Pharmaceuticals. Griggs became interested in Obetrol and therefore acquired the company. He asked one simple question: *Could the United States, with its notoriously short memory, be ready to try amphetamine again? Of course, it would, with the right marketing.*

Griggs acquired Rexar and started marketing Obetrol with a new brand name. It is interesting to know how Griggs arrived at the brand name. He acquired Rexar suspecting that Obetrol might treat ADHD, even without testing, because a pediatrician in Utah prescribed much of it for ADHD. Also, he knew that ADHD was found in 3 to 5 percent of the children at the time. So it was indeed a significant opportunity. *He took 'ADD' (from Attention Deficit Disorder) and fiddled with some suffixes: All for ADD, ADD for All - Adderall!* Griggs later recalled that it was meant to be a kind of inclusive thing.

He went ahead and marketed Adderall for ADHD without FDA approval. The drug was not even tested for its efficacy in treating the condition. FDA very soon halted the marketing of the drug. In response, Richmond Pharmaceuticals started a trial and submitted a new drug application (NDA). The company was unsure whether the FDA would approve its application. As luck would have it, Griggs received a phone call from a well-connected Washington lobbyist, who told him that a US senator was furious that his son could no longer obtain Adderall. And sure enough, the FDA approved the Adderall new drug application. Later, Griggs sold his company, Richwood Pharmaceuticals, to Shire Pharmaceuticals. Shire marketed both ADHD and Adderall with equal vigor.

Shire Markets ADHD and Adderall Aggressively

Shire spared no effort in marketing the ADHD condition with its key brand Adderall. It conducted disease awareness and education campaigns, engaged multiple stakeholders, and heavily advertised in print and television. It also had a considerable online presence through its websites for information and education of teachers, parents, and healthcare professionals. Here are some of the important marketing and advertising initiatives that the company has been taking over the years:

- Gathered hundreds of doctors at many company-sponsored meetings, where a specialist physician (child psychiatrist or child psychologist of repute) paid by the company explained the value of Adderall in treating ADHD.
- Massive personal selling effort to engage physicians frequently with communication inputs, such as posters, visual-aids highlighting the benefits like better grades and behavior that Adderall could offer. Shire representatives used to visit at the time all psychiatrists in their respective areas once every two weeks to promote Adderall.

- Sponsored ADHD patient advocacy groups such as CHADD (Children and Adults with ADHD) to spread awareness of the condition.
- Has been sponsoring online ADHD self-assessment tests to drive diagnoses. Shire sponsored, for example, a quiz. Could *you have ADHD?* On the website, everydayhealth.com, Shire advertised the quiz sometime in 2011, featuring the celebrity singer Levine of Maroon 5, which resulted in about 570,000 people taking the test, according to Medical Marketing & Media.
- Partnered with TV personality Ty Pennington, a popular television host, and later Maroon 5 star Adam Levine to spread awareness of Adult ADHD in their campaign, *It's your ADHD - Own it.*
- Sponsored a medical education video portraying a physician diagnosing the disorder in an adult in a six-minute conversation, after which the doctor recommends the medication.
- Shire once subsidized 50,000 copies of a comic book that tries to demystify the disorder and uses Superheroes to tell children *that medication may make it easier to pay attention and control their behavior.*
- Shire paid CHADD, the ADHD advocacy group, $3 million from 2006 to 2009 to have the group's bi-monthly magazine, *Attention*, distributed to doctors' offices nationwide.
- Shire also targeted parents in its Direct-to-consumer advertisements. The company carried a wrap-around advertisement for Adderall XR on the People magazine cover of September 2005, which showed a mother hugging her smiling child, holding a sheet of paper with a "B+" written. The advertisement read— *Finally! School work that matches her intelligence.*
- Shire designed compelling advertising messages, even if misleading, based on Dr. Joseph Biederman's (a prominent child psychiatrist at Harvard) studies it sponsored. One of the advertisements says: *Adderall XR improves academic performance*.

Attention Continues

That is a brief account of how attention deficit hyperactivity disorder (ADHD) has evolved and continues to grow. Recently a few non-stimulant drugs too have entered the market. These are—Straterra (atomoxetine) by Eli Lilly, and Kapvay (clonidine) by Shionogi.

The two major players primarily responsible for the phenomenal growth of ADHD are Ritalin of Novartis, and Adderall of Shire Pharmaceuticals. Ritalin started it all in 1956, and Adderall took the mantle once Ritalin lost its market exclusivity. Ritalin has been an enduring brand in treating the condition for over sixty years. Methylphenidate (Ritalin and many other brands of methylphenidate) continues to play an essential role in treating ADHD. And the sixty-plus Methylphenidate, a senior citizen of the ADHD-medication community, is still fit as a fiddle!

(Source: Adapted from articles— 1. Adam Gaffney, How ADHD was sold, The New Republic, September 23, 2016, 2. Vincent Iannelli, MD, A history of medication timeline of ADHD, VeryWell Mind, September 05, 2018, www.verywellmind.com; 3. ADHD History, www.adhd-brain.com)

CASE

39

Requip's Success Recipe: Brand A Disease, Market A Treatment!

Karl A. Ekborn, a Swedish neurologist, first described a condition known as Ekborn's Syndrome in the mid-1940s. The syndrome is characterized by sensory symptoms and motor disturbances in the limbs during rest. Earlier descriptions of such a condition date back to the 17th century. Thomas Willis, the English anatomist and physician from 1621 to 1675, first described these symptoms. Restless Legs Syndrome is the new name for Ekborn syndrome. National Institute of Neurological Disorders and Stroke at NIH (National Institutes of Health) describes restless legs syndrome (RLS) as:

RLS is a neurological disorder characterized by unpleasant sensations in the legs and an uncontrollable urge to move when at rest to relieve these feelings. The sensations are described as burning, creeping, tugging, or like insects crawling inside the legs. These sensations are known as abnormal (paresthesias) or unpleasant (dysesthesias) in medical literature.

GlaxoSmithKline's (GSK) marketing of Requip offers a classic example of disease branding. Requip (ropinirole) is a drug used for treating Parkinson's Disease. GSK found the drug is also useful in treating a little-known condition called Restless Legs Syndrome (RLS). As a result, FDA approved Requip for the treatment of RLS in 2005.

Clinicians saw Restless Legs Syndrome (RLS) until a few years ago, till GSK started its awareness campaigns, as an unusual, somewhat mysterious condition. It was characterized by a crawling sensation in the legs, often more severe at night, which could be relieved by movement such as walking. It was not a common affliction. Not until GSK got approval from the FDA for its Requip in treating RLS. Getting approval for your drug for a lesser known, infrequently occurring condition is one thing; marketing a drug profitably for that condition is quite another.

How do you market your drug, although approved for treating a little-known condition? GSK thought out a clear-cut strategy. The strategy of creating a market for this little-known, under-diagnosed, and under-treated condition is called RLS. GSK, the second largest pharmaceutical company at the time in the world, made good use of public relations and its marketing muscle to promote awareness among doctors and patients about RLS.

GSK started its awareness campaigns on Restless Legs Syndrome months before FDA's approval in medical journals targeting doctors. However, on getting the approval for Requip, Glaxo soon issued a press release titled, "*New survey reveals common yet under-recognized disorder — restless legs syndrome — is keeping Americans awake at night!*" The Requip public relations campaign suggested that problems such as insomnia and depression might be symptoms of restless legs syndrome, which tormented as many as one in ten Americans.

After the public awareness campaign and the FDA approval, Requip experienced substantial growth. In the process, the company created a blue ocean that it was expected to own for a long time.

However, GSK's marketing effort and its initial success for Requip in RLS had drawn criticism from various quarters. Critics felt that RLS was a concocted disorder and that the company had resorted to disease mongering to promote the sale of the drug. There was also some criticism that GSK's marketing of RLS had many conflicts of interest, such as using patient advocacy groups (PAGs) and key opinion leaders (KOLs) to further its marketing agenda.

The NBC Nightly News aired on January 31, 2007, a story on Restless Legs Syndrome disorder and why GlaxoSmithKline, the world's second-largest pharmaceutical company, had so heavily advertised its drug, Requip (Ropinirole hydrochloride) for this disorder on the news channel. Some critics viewed this as a mere publicity stunt. However, the RLS disorder, perceived as an uncommon condition, soon became a household name after GSK started its marketing effort to increase public awareness.

GSK also started direct-to-consumer advertising (DTCA) campaigns after the FDA approved Requip for RLS. Initial ads were brand awareness advertisements and unbranded campaigns. These were later followed up with branded ads.

GSK also used key opinion leaders (KOLs) such as sleep specialists to raise awareness about RLS and its scope for Requip among general practitioners (GPs). In addition, the company's overall marketing efforts in raising awareness through multiple channels got a lot of media attention, creating publicity for the disorder (RLS) and the drug (Requip).

The Wall Street Journal commented on the overall marketing efforts and success of Requip in 2006 when it stated: *Behind Requip's sales boom is Glaxo's marketing machine, which has persuaded many consumers and physicians to accept restless legs syndrome, or RLS, as a real condition warranting treatment*.

Besides criticism, GSK's marketing efforts also got praise from some quarters, such as marketing experts, doctors, and patient advocacy groups. They particularly appreciated the unbranded campaigns that strove to increase awareness about the disease. In addition, some doctors and patient advocates praised GSK for raising the profile of the disorder, which was under-diagnosed and under-treated.

How did restless legs and Reequip happen? GlaxoSmithKline believed that Requip held much promise in treating restless legs syndrome. It hit upon the idea of marketing Requip for RLS after observing that some doctors were prescribing the drug off-label to treat this condition, RLS. On March 31, 2003, GSK started the RLS promotion with press releases about a research paper presented at the 55th American Academy of Neurology (AAN) meetings in Honolulu, which described the early results of using ropinirole for the treatment of RLS. FDA approved Requip, and marketing blitz followed approval. GSK had put all its marketing might behind Requip in RLS through multichannel marketing, involving personal selling, CMEs by KOLs and thought leaders, and unbranded and branded DTC campaigns targeting all key stakeholders such as doctors, patients, and payers.

What are the results of all this marketing effort behind Requip? First, the company observed that the number of patients treated for RLS grew from 3,80, 000 in 2006, to 2.2 million in 2015. The market size for this little-known condition or disorder in 2005 had also increased from a few million dollars to US $1.7 billion by 2015.

GSK's response to all the negative criticism, such as disease mongering and conflict of interest about its marketing of Requip was best summed up by David Stout, Head of Pharmaceuticals, GlaxoSmithKline Plc, when he said: *You need to talk to the patients. Things like restless legs syndrome can ruin people's lives. It is easy to trivialize things when you don't have them. If people did not want the treatment, they would not seek them.*

With GlaxoSmithKline's marketing might and a firm conviction of its effectiveness behind it, Requip ran on its Restless Legs (syndrome)!

(Source: Adapted from— Rajiv Fernando and Debapratim Purkaystha, GlaxoSmithKline's Marketing Strategy for Requip: A Case Study in Product Lifecycle Management, IBS Center for Management Research published in 2007)

CASE

40

Pfizer, PSTD, and Zoloft!

In 1980, the American Psychiatric Association added post-traumatic stress disorder (PTSD) to the third edition of its Diagnostic and Statistical Manual of Mental Disorders (DSM). PTSD, primarily, almost exclusively, had been associated with combat veterans and victims of violent crime. However, Pfizer set out in 1999 to change that, convincing Americans that PTSD could afflict almost anyone after getting the US FDA's approval for its Zoloft (sertraline) in treating PTSD.

Pfizer had left no stone unturned in raising awareness for PTSD. Here are some of its more significant actions in this regard:

1. Pfizer funded the creation of the PTSD Alliance and staffed it with its public relations firm, The Chandler Chicco Agency, which ran it from its offices.
2. One of the essential functions of the alliance was to build a network of journalists and thought leaders in PTSD. The alliance connected mainstream media journalists with PTSD experts like Jerilyn Ross, President, and CEO of Anxiety Disorders Association of America, whom the Pharma majors such as Pfizer and GlaxoSmithKline heavily subsidized.
3. Shortly after Zoloft's campaign in PTSD, media mentions of PTSD grew substantially. The New York Times, for example, ran a story with statistics provided by Pfizer on childhood

PTSD, quoting that minors who experience the sudden death of a close friend or a relative will develop the disorder. Even other papers and magazines carried articles highlighting the studies promoted by the alliance. The studies indicated that 1 in 13 Americans would have PTSD at some point in time.

4. On September 26, 2001, The PTSD Alliance stated from its office at Pfizer's PR firm, Chandler Chicco, that post-traumatic stress can affect anyone who has witnessed a violent act or experienced natural disasters or other unexpected catastrophic or psychologically distressing events, such as September 11 terrorist attacks.
5. In October 2001, Pfizer had spent US $5.6 million, 25 percent more than its average ad spending per month, on advertising Zoloft's benefits in treating PTSD.

Pfizer's massive public relations effort, combined with its promotion to physicians, significantly passed the US $2.3 billion mark in Zoloft's annual sales.

(Adapted from Article: Brendan I. Koerner, *Disorders Made to Order*, Mother Jones, July/August 2002)

CASE

41

Merck Creates A Market for A Bone Disease, Fields Its New Drug, Fosamax And Makes it the Market Leader!

Merck had in-licensed an early stage new chemical compound alendronate (Fosamax) in 1988 from Instituto Gentili, an Italian pharmaceutical and biotechnology company, for further development and commercialization. The company obtained US FDA approval for Fosamax, a first-in-class (bisphosphonates) compound for the treatment of Osteoporosis, in 1995.

Osteoporosis has been a serious problem affecting millions of women. Therefore, the potential market for Fosamax was enormous. Fosamax could become a blockbuster drug. However, the problem was Fosamax had a very poor sales uptake in the first two years. The company came up with a three-pronged strategy:

1. Expanding diagnosis
2. Obtaining multiple indications
3. Developing new formulations

Expanding Diagnosis

How Merck expanded diagnosis is an exciting story involving some out-of-the-box thinking. However, before that, a brief overview of the market scenario surrounding Osteoporosis at the time.

Osteoporosis is a disease that causes bones to become brittle and break more easily. It mostly affects older women, and a fall can be devastating with breaking a hip. One in five older women who break a hip will die within a year.

Osteopenia is different from Osteoporosis. Think of it as a midpoint between having healthy bones and Osteoporosis. WEB MD says that Osteopenia is when your bones are weaker than normal but not so far gone that they break easily, which is the hallmark of Osteoporosis. Your bones are usually at their densest when you are about thirty. Osteopenia, if it happens at all, often occurs after age fifty.

Osteopenia is also the story of how the definition of what constitutes a disease evolves and the role that drug companies can play in that evolution.

Osteopenia as a condition was hardly known in the early 1990s. Only a handful of people would have heard even about the word—Osteopenia. Merck's strategy of expanding the diagnosis had played a significant role in transforming Osteopenia from the status of a rarely heard word into a diagnosis for which millions of women swallow pills to slow the progress of the condition further to Osteoporosis. The whole process of diagnosing Osteopenia began at a meeting of a group of renowned experts on Osteoporosis in 1992 in Rome, under the auspices of the World Health Organization (WHO), to arrive at a consensus on diagnosing and measuring Osteoporosis. The group of experts created a category of Osteopenia mostly because they thought it might be useful for public health researchers who like clear categories for their studies. They never thought that people would come to think of Osteopenia as a disease in itself to be treated when they created it!

How did Osteopenia transform from a category for public health researchers to a condition that millions of women want to get treated for? That brings us to Jeremy Allen, the man who measured the bone.

Jeremy Allen retired from IMS Health, an American company engaged in providing healthcare information and technology to the healthcare industry worldwide, in 1991, and set up a consulting business in the US. In 1995, he was approached by David Anstice, the president of Merck. The latter was also his former colleague at IMS Health before he took the position at Merck, with a proposition: *Fosamax, the first-in-class drug for Osteoporosis with tremendous market potential, was not getting enough prescriptions and sales. Figure out this problem and fix it.*

How you generate more prescriptions for Fosamax seemed an obvious question. Get more diagnoses. How do you get more diagnoses of Osteoporosis? More bone scans, of course!

However, in 1995, there was just no way of getting more scans done in America. The machines that measured bone density were scarce. There were only huge tabletop machines to measure bone density, and the scans cost between $200 to $350 per test. Besides, there were just a couple of hundred testing centers across the US, which made it even more difficult to access.

To sell Fosamax, Merck had to increase the number of scans because no diagnosis was possible without a bone densitometry test. To expand diagnosis, the company had to do two things:

1. Place machines that could measure bone density in doctors' offices across America, and
2. Bring down the price of bone scans

Merck and Allen had gone about changing how the American Healthcare system measured bone to achieve these two objectives. First, they started Bone Measurement Institute, a non-profit organization, to serve the public good. Although six of the most respected Osteoporosis researchers were on its board, the Institute was essentially a one-person show with Allen as its sole employee. His desk at Merck's office was the office of the Institute too.

Merck needed smaller, more affordable, and even portable machines to measure bone density so that doctors could do the tests in their offices. These machines were called peripheral machines, and they measured the bone density in the forearm, heel, wrist, or fingers than the hip and spine. Few manufacturers made these peripheral machines as the demand was low because they did not measure the hip and spine. However, these machines were the perfect fit for Merck's strategy, which aims to keep as many machines as needed in doctors' offices and to reduce the cost of bone scans. In addition, being small, they would not take up much office space and cost only a fraction of the big central machines.

Merck started a campaign to increase the manufacture and promotion of peripheral machines. The company even took an equity position in a company to begin manufacturing the peripheral machines, essentially to demonstrate its strategic intent. However, the big dominant players who manufactured the huge central machines that measured the hip and spine were hostile to these peripheral machines. There was also criticism and resistance to the peripheral machines stating that it was not a good basis for diagnosis and would lead to bad medicine.

However, Merck was hellbent on taking up the cause of spreading the peripheral machines and making the prices of bone density tests affordable. So Merck bought one of the companies that manufactured peripheral machines and showed how low the price could become, primarily to get everyone's attention. Moreover, to prove that peripheral machines were not inferior, Merck took the position that the peripheral bone density scans had a good correlation in providing adequate information about the risk of hip and spine fractures and backed it by many studies. Furthermore, Merck partnered with diagnostic equipment manufacturers Hologic and Lunar corporations to finance the rollout of bone-mineral testing machines even in far-flung areas that are thinly populated.

Strategic Lobbying

Merck worked hard to get the smaller machines into doctors' offices and did not stop with that. Merck funded the required trials and helped peripheral machines with submissions to get through the FDA process. Merck also conducted massive education campaigns about the availability of new, inexpensive peripheral machines. For example, the Fosamax sales force distributed promotional literature highlighting these machines' usage and prices to doctors during their visits. Furthermore, Merck created a leasing program so that doctors could finance a large or small machine purchase.

The Birth of A Diagnosis

Perhaps Merck's most important and notable strategic move was to change the economics of measuring the bone reimbursable by Medicare. In 1997, the Bone Measurement Institute and other interested organizations successfully lobbied to pass the Bone Measurement Act, legislation that changed Medicare reimbursement rules to cover bone scans. Merck funded several organizations that have lobbied for the bill.

As a matter of strategic coincidence, in 1997, Merck got clearance from the FDA for a new lower dose of Fosamax, a 5-milligram tablet for those women diagnosed with Osteopenia. Merck helped place most of the machines in doctors' offices across the US. The ease of diagnosis and the new legislation that made bone scans reimbursable expanded the diagnosis of Osteopenia and Osteoporosis phenomenally. The new peripheral machines made the diagnosis so simple that they generated a report with three distinct colors: Green, Yellow, and Red; Green meant normal, Yellow meant Osteopenia, and Red indicated Osteoporosis.

The very mention of the word Osteopenia on a report and the color-coded diagnosis profoundly affected millions of women that it was a disease. So when you have a condition, you should get it treated, and there is treatment now for Osteopenia. So you can maintain bone health with that.

In addition, Merck ran commercials advertising drugs to prevent Osteoporosis. Interestingly, those commercials didn't feature humped grannies but young-looking women. In addition, the focus was on Osteopenia, which had a larger patient pool. Finally, through testing and advertising, a cultural consensus took hold. Osteopenia became a condition that was seriously considered for treatment. A diagnosis was born!

Proof of the Pudding

Merck's efforts to expand diagnoses of Osteoporosis and Osteopenia were a phenomenal success. However, the proof of the pudding is in the eating. Consider these statistics:

- Medicare claims for bone scanning exams increased from 77,000 in 1994 to more than 1.5 million annually by 1997. The New Medicare benefit was standardized in 1998.
- The sale of peripheral machines increased more than 500 percent over the same period. The Bone Densitometry centers had grown from 2000 in 1995 to 7,500 in a short period.
- The cost of a bone measuring test dropped to less than $30 per test from over $200.
- Fosamax became a blockbuster with $1.04 billion in 1999. It took close to four years for Fosamax to achieve its first billion-dollar mark. It reached over $2 billion in annual sales in 2002 and $3.2 billion by 2004.

Multiple Indications

Merck had also obtained approval for three new indications in addition to the initial 1995 approval of Postmenopausal Osteoporosis (PMO) treatment of (10 mg) and Paget's disease (40 mg). The details of the new indications are presented in the following table.

Table 2.3 Fosamax Indication Approvals

New Indication Approval by the US FDA	Date of Approval
PMO Prevention 5 mg (Osteopenia)	2nd Quarter, 1997
Glucocorticoid-induced Osteoporosis (5/10mg)	3rd Quarter, 1999
Male Osteoporosis (10mg)	4th Quarter, 2000

New Formulations

The most effective growth strategy of Fosamax had been the development of a once-weekly Fosamax formulation of 35/70 mg. The FDA approved it in November 2000. It had the same price as the daily tablets and immediately cannibalized the sales of the regular formula. However, It had grown overall sales of Fosamax. Fosamax once weekly was a breakaway success taking more than 80 percent of franchise sales within the first two years. The gastrointestinal side effects present with the daily dose had considerably eased with the once-weekly formulation of Fosamax. The original molecule patent expired in 2008, and the Fosamax OW (once-weekly) formula patent would be valid until 2018.

Fosamax Once-weekly thus had the power to prevent the generic erosion to no small extent. Besides, on April 17, 2005, Merck gained FDA approval for a Fixed-Dose-Combination (FDC) of alendronate sodium plus cholecalciferol (Vitamin D3) under the brand name Fosamax Plus D for the treatment of Osteoporosis in postmenopausal women and to increase bone mass in men. Fosamax Plus D too helped Merck to consolidate its osteoporosis franchise.

Effective Lifecycle Management

Merck had managed the Fosamax timeline well despite challenges. It had launched new indications and formulations well before patent expiry. It had its share of challenges, such as:

- Low diagnosis and treatment rates
- Low long-term compliance

- Low Franchise equity in women's health
- Delayed consumer marketing opportunity to raise awareness (Branded DTC advertising did not start till 2001)

At the same time, Merck also had a big opportunity when the doubts were cast on Hormonal Replacement Therapy for menopausal women. Merck seized the opportunity with its DTC advertising. It also increased the sales force's emphasis on obstetric and gynecology therapeutic areas.

Merck did exceedingly well in developing the Osteoporosis market and creating a condition called Osteopenia out of virtually nowhere. In addition, Merck did an excellent job of maintaining its dominance within the bisphosphonates class.

Lessons

Merck created a market for bone disease remarkably, expanded the market through increased awareness, fielded a drug to treat it, and even made it a market leader. However, Merck did not create an enduring osteoporosis franchise, the disorder that it expanded so dramatically. Here are the key lessons:

1. *Identify the unmet needs and shape your market around them*. Merck identified a substantial unmet need in Osteoporosis and Osteopenia. Osteopenia was unheard of before Merck began its awareness programs and campaigns.
2. *Begin your market-shaping activity long before the launch*. Most brand teams start their marketing activities months before the launch. The most effective companies begin the market shaping work during the clinical development work once they see the initial promise of the drug to transform both the disease perception and the product profile long before launch. Merck invested in an intensive campaign to educate physicians (gynecologists mainly) and the American public (especially middle-aged women) about Osteoporosis and the availability of bone-mineral testing. Merck's efforts expanded the potential

market from 1.3 million per year in the US to 16 million women at risk in a short period.

3. *Involve and engage as many stakeholders as necessary* to raise awareness of the disease condition and how the product is best suited to treat it. Merck co-sponsored media campaigns with the National Osteoporosis Foundation.
4. *Go beyond conventional partnerships* such as patient advocacy groups and physicians to meet unmet needs. For Fosamax, Merck partnered with diagnostic equipment manufacturers Hologic and Lunar corporations to finance the rollout of bone-mineral testing machines in far-flung, sparsely populated areas.
5. *Expand indications and develop new formulations* to extend market exclusivity and patient segments, increasing short, and long-term sales.
6. *Improving access and insurance coverage* are vital to make your new drug a blockbuster. Merck worked hard to bring down the prices of bone scans. The company, along with other organizations, got legislation, the Bone Measurement Act, that makes bone scans reimbursable.

(Source: Adapted from Alix Spiegel's article, *How a bone disease grew to fit the prescription*, NPR, December 21, 2009; and *Building Global Bio brands: Taking biotechnology to market*, by Francois Simmons and Philip Kotler)

CHAPTER

3

Drug Repositioning

The most fruitful basis of the discovery of the new drug is to start with an old drug.

—*James Black, a Physician, and Pharmacologist, shared the 1988 Nobel Prize for Medicine for pioneering rational drug-design strategies, leading to Propranolol and Cimetidine.*

Drug Repositioning

Drug Repositioning by Repurposing Drugs

Drug Repurposing (DR) is also known by several other terms, such as drug repositioning, drug-re-tasking, drug profiling, drug rescuing, drug recycling, drug redirection, and therapeutic switching. However, this definition of drug repurposing has been extended later to include active substances that failed in the clinical phase of their development due to their toxicity, insufficient efficacy, and drugs called back from the market due to safety concerns.

Drug repurposing is a process of identification of new pharmacological indications from old/existing/failed/already marketed/pro-drugs, and investigational new drugs being developed for the treatment of diseases other than the drug's original, or intended therapeutic use. Compared to the high costs, a long time to develop, and high risk of failure associated with drug discovery programs, drug repurposing takes relatively lesser time, has lower costs, and has a low risk of failure. Therefore, many pharmaceutical companies actively pursue drug repurposing to introduce new products.

The Drug repositioning trend, which is the use of a drug in an indication than the one for which it was initially marketed, is growing. For example, according to recent estimates, the market for repurposed drugs grew from $24.4 billion in 2015 to $31.3 billion in 2020.

The first drug repositioning in the 1920s was an accidental discovery based on serendipitous observations. Later, pharmaceutical scientists developed more approaches to accelerate drug repurposing. The key drivers of this growth in drug repositioning are the advancement of bioinformatics, availability of huge biological and structural databases, which have significantly reduced the time and cost of drug development, and the risk of failure.

Drug Repurposing: Two Approaches

Drug repositioning has two alternative approaches—one is an experiment-based approach, and the other is *in silico*-based approach.

The experiment-based approach is also known as activity-based repositioning, which refers to the screening of original drugs for new pharmacological indications based on experimental assays.

***In Silico* approach** to repositioning, on the other hand, carries out virtual screening of public databases of huge drug and chemical libraries using computational biology and bioinformatics, and chemoinformatic tools. In this approach, researchers identify potential bioactive molecules based on the molecular interaction between drug molecules and protein targets.

Here is a table summarizing the differences between activity—and *in-silico-based* approaches to drug repositioning.

Table 3.1 Differences Between Activity-Based and In Silico-Based Approaches in Drug Repositioning

Activity-Based Approach	*In Silico*-Based Approach
Experimental (*in vitro* and *in vivo* screening)	Computational (virtual) screening
Target-based and cell/organism-based screening assay	Protein target-based screening
Requires no structural information of target proteins and drug-induced cell/disease phenotypic information	Requires structural information of target proteins and drug-induced cell/disease phenotypic information
Time and labor consuming	Time and labor efficient
Lower rate of false positive hits during the screening	Higher rate of false positive hits during the screening

(Source: Mithun Rajpal, Shubham J. Khairnar, and Anil G. Jadhav, Drug Repurposing (DR): An Emerging Approach in Drug Discovery, **intechopen.com**, April 26, 2020)

The in silico approach has been increasingly popular over the past few decades, with significant success in drug discovery programs. It offers significant advantages such as reduced development time and cost and a low risk of failure.

Two Main Strategies

Mithun Rudrapal, Shubham J. Khairnar, and Anil G. Jadhav explain the strategies and approaches to drug repurposing in a chapter they wrote—*Drug Repurposing (DR): An Emerging Approach in Drug Discovery* for a book, Drug Repurposing edited by Farid A. Badria. This chapter was published on intechopen.com on April 26, 2020. Here is the gist: The strategies of drug repurposing (DR) are—on-target, and off-target.

On-target drug repurposing is applying the known pharmacological mechanism of a drug molecule to a new therapeutic indication. In this strategy, the biological target of the molecule is the same, but the disease is different. For example, in the repositioning of minoxidil (Rogaine), an on-target profile indicated that the drug produces two different therapeutic effects while acting on the same target. As an antihypertensive vasodilator, minoxidil widens the blood vessels and opens potassium channels, allowing more oxygen, blood, and nutrients to the hair follicles. This pharmacological action helps its use in treating male pattern baldness (androgenic alopecia).

Off-target drug repurposing, on the other hand, the pharmacological mechanism is unknown. In addition, drugs and drug candidates act on new targets beyond the original scope for new therapeutic indications. Therefore, both the targets and the indications are new. Aspirin (Colsprin) is a good example of an off-target profile. Aspirin, apart from its known for its anti-inflammatory, analgesic, and antipyretic properties, also suppresses blood coagulation (clot formation) by inhibiting the normal functioning of platelets (anti-platelet action). It is, therefore, used in treating heart attacks and strokes. More recently, Aspirin's use in the treatment of prostate cancer is also being studied.

Big Opportunity

The Drug Repurposing online website, drugrepurposing.info , has a huge database of 9,040 compounds that have been either launched, registered, or investigated, covering 475 indications with 1,021 mechanisms. With 3,107 links between mechanism and indications, 844 links between compound and indication, and 279 links between compound and mechanism (off-target effects), drug repurposing offers 4,230 repurposing opportunities, and that is huge!

Table 3.2 Repositioned Drugs: Some Examples

Drug	Original Indication	New Indication
Amphotericin B (AMB), Anti-fungal antibiotic	Fungal infections	Leishmaniasis
Aspirin, NSAID	Pain and inflammation	Cardio Vascualar (Anti-platelet activity)
Aspirin, NSAID	Pain and inflammation	Prostate cancer (under development)
Amantadine, Anti-viral)	Influenza	Parkinson's Disease
Atomoxetine, Anti-depressant	Depression	ADHD (Attention Deficit Hyperactivity Disorder
Bupropion, SSRI, Anti-depressant	Depression	Smoking Cessation
Crizotinib	Lymphoma (under clinical trial for Ana-plastic large cell lymphoma)	Non-small cell lung cancer (Already developed)
Colchicine, Anti-inflammatory agent	Gout (Gouty arthritis)	Pericarditis
Daunorubicin, Chemotherapeutic agent	Acute myeloid leukemia (AML) and Acute lymphoblastic leukemia (ALL)	Breast cancer
Dimethyl fumarate, Anti-allergic	Psoriasis	Multiple Sclerosis (MS)
Dimethyl fumarate, Anti-allergic	Psoriasis	Multiple Sclerosis (MS)
Duloxetine, SSNRI	Depression	General Anxiety Disorder (GAD), Fibromyalgia, Chronic musculoskeletal pain, neuropathic pain
Everolimus, Immune suppressant	Immune suppressant	Pancreatic neuroendocrine tumors

Table 3.2 *Contd...*

Drug	Original Indication	New Indication
Fluorouracil, Antimetabolite, Anti-cancer	Cancer	Breast cancer
Gabapentin, Anti-epileptic	Epilepsy	Neuropathic pain
Galantamine, AChE (Acetylcho-linesterase) inhibitor	Neuromuscular paralysis	Alzheimer's Disease (AD)
Ibudilast, PDE (Phospho-diesterase) inhibitor	Asthma	Neuropathic pain
Imatinib, TKI (Tyrosin Kinase Inhibitors), Anti-cancer	CML (Chronic Myelogenous Leukemia), ALL (Acute Lymphoblastic Leukemia)	GIST (Gastrointestinal Stromal Tumor)
Isoniazid, Anti-tubercular	Tuberculosis	Certain types of tumor
Methotrexate, Anti-metabolite (Anti-cancer)	Cancer	Psoriasis, Rheumatoid Arthritis (RA)
Mifepristone, Antiprogestin	Termination of pregnancy in combination with misoprostol	Cushing syndrome
Minoxidil, Vasodilator (Antihypertensive)	Hypertension	Androgenic alopecia
Orlistat, Anti-obesity agent	Obesity	Cancer
Propranolol, Beta Blocker	Hypertension	Migraine
Ropinrole, Anti-Parkinson's drug	Parkinson's Disease (PD)	Restless leg syndrome (RLS)
Sildenafil, PDE (Phospho-diesterase) inhibitor	Angina pectoris, Pulmonary arterial hypertension	Erectile dysfunction (ED)

Table 3.2 *Contd...*

Drug	Original Indication	New Indication
Simvastatin, Hypolipidemic	CVDs (Cardiovascular Disorders)	Lung cancer
Sunitinib, TKI (Ani-cancer)	Imatinib-resistant GIST, RCC (Renal cell carcinoma)	Pancreatic neuroendocrine tumors
Tamoxifen, Anti-cancer	Breast cancer, Anti-cancer	Systemic lupus erthmatosus
Thalidomide, Immune modulator	Immuno-modulation, Morning sickness (withdrawn)	Multiple myeloma, Leprosy
Topiramate	Partial onset of seizures, Primary generalized tonic-clonic seizures	Migraine
Valproic acid, Anti-epileptic	Epilepsy	Maniac depression (Bi-polar disorder), Migraine headache
Zidovudine, Anti-viral	Cancer (failed clinical trial)	HIV (Human Immunodeficiency Virus), AIDS (Acquired Immunodeficiency Syndrome)

(Source: Mithun Rajpal, Shubham J. Khairnar, and Anil G. Jadhav, Drug Repurposing (DR): An Emerging Approach in Drug Discovery, **intechopen.com**, April 26, 2020)

The following cases present some notable examples of drug repositioning by repurposing already approved drugs.

CASE

42

Aspirin at 120: Not Retired, But Repurposed!

Aspirin (acetylsalicylic acid) is the first-ever drug to be repurposed.

In 1899, Bayer, the global drug major from Germany, marketed Aspirin first as an analgesic. Later in 1980, Aspirin was repositioned as an anti-platelet aggregation drug to prevent cardiovascular events, such as myocardial infarction and stroke, in low doses. Dr. Lawrence Craven, a suburban general practitioner in Glendale, California, first reported this antithrombic effect of Aspirin. In 1950, Dr. Craven published his first letter in the *Annals of Western Medicine and Surgery*, in which he introduced his hypothesis that Aspirin was preventive for coronary thrombosis. He cited evidence that Aspirin prolonged prothrombin time and mentioned reports of more frequent hemorrhaging among patients who chewed Aspirin gum after a tonsillectomy or a tooth extraction.

Aspirin's usage in the second indication as an antithrombotic agent began much later based on Dr. John R. Vane's work, for which he received the Nobel Prize for Medicine in 1982.

Aspirin may soon be repositioned again, this time in oncology. Research studies show that daily administration of Aspirin for at least five years can prevent the development of many cancers, particularly colorectal cancer. However, although this second repositioning of Aspirin offers great promise, the pharmaceutical industry may not seem keen due to the difficulties in navigating the maze of intellectual property issues.

(Source: Adapted from articles—1. Jonathan Miner, BS, BA, and Adam Hoffhines, BS, The Discovery of Aspirin's Antithrombotic Effects, Texas Heart Institute Journal, 2007, 34 (2): 179-186, 2. Jean-Pierre Jourdan, Ronan Bureau, Christophe Rochais, Patrick Dallemagne, Drug Positioning: A Brief Overview, Journal of Pharmacy and Pharmacology / Volume 72, Issue 9/ p. 1145-1151, Wiley Online Library.com)

CASE

43

A Banned Drug Gets Repositioned for the Second Time!

In 1957, Grunenthal, a West German pharmaceutical company, first launched Thalidomide as a sedative for a sleepless post-World War Europe. An accidental discovery revealed that the drug also cures nausea. Soon, doctors worldwide started prescribing Thalidomide to pregnant women for morning sickness. Unfortunately, the babies of these women who were taking Thalidomide for morning sickness were tragically born with congenital deformities, such as shortened or completely absent limbs. The manufacturers failed to detect these harmful effects in their animal studies. In 1962, the World Health Organization (WHO) banned Thalidomide due to its teratogenicity, affecting thousands of victims worldwide.

Despite the ban, in 1964, Dr. Jacob Sheskin from Hadassah University, Jerusalem, demonstrated Thalidomide's dramatic efficacy against erythema nodosum leprosum, an autoimmune complication of leprosy, a rare disease with an estimated incidence of 250,000 cases per year. Later, In 1998, Celgene (part of Bristol-Myers Squibb, now) repositioned Thalidomide as an orphan drug for complications of leprosy. Celgene's repositioning of Thalidomide illustrates that you can reposition drugs, even with an exceptionally high toxicity profile, if the new indication is a rare disease.

In addition, Thalidomide has been repositioned like Aspirin for the second time in oncology. Thalidomide's teratogenicity demonstrated its antiangiogenic activity, which is responsible for the arrested limb development (phocomelia) that occurs after *in-utero* exposure leading to further research into its potential use to block or destroy blood vessels supplying blood to malignant tumors. In 2006, the US FDA lifted the ban on Thalidomide and allowed limited distribution to treat leprosy and multiple myeloma, a cancer of plasma cells.

After being taken off the market in 1962, Thalidomide made a comeback in several countries a few years ago. Consider these, for example:

- Dabur India Limited got approval from Central Drugs Standard Control Organization to market it for the treatment of leprosy in India in 2002.
- Japan allowed its use for cancer treatment in 2008.
- Thalidomide was made available in Brazil, too, a few years back.

Scientists are hopeful of safer Thalidomide versions in the future. Suvro Chatterjee of Anna University, Chennai, India, says: *When the drug's binding target is known, avenues open to engineer the molecule for better action*.

(Source: Adapted from articles—1. Dinsa Sachan, The Thalidomide Story Explained, downtoearth.com, April 30, 2010, 2. Jean-Pierre Jourdan, Ronan Bureau, Christophe Rochais, Patrick Dallemagne, Drug Positioning: A Brief Overview, Journal of Pharmacy and Pharmacology / Volume 72, Issue 9/ p. 1145-1151, Wiley Online Library.com)

CASE

44

Revatio, Viagra's New Avatar!

In the late 1980s and 1990s, Pfizer developed sildenafil, the active ingredient in Viagra, originally to treat angina, a form of chest pain caused by limited blood flow to the heart muscles. However, an unexpected side effect emerged during the clinical trials in the UK in the form of penile erections. It acts by inhibiting phosphodiesterase type-5 (PDE5) enzyme, which leads to vasodilation and consequently blocks cGMP (Cyclic Guanosine Monophosphate) degradation. So, what does this mean? PDE5 is an enzyme in the smooth muscle cells of your blood vessels. Its specific function within your body is complex, but at a basic level, PDE5 helps control the blood flow through blood vessels in certain body parts. It does this by causing your blood vessels to constrict. So, when sildenafil inhibits PDE5, your blood vessels become larger, letting more blood flow to certain types of tissue, thus helping to get and maintain an erection.

As a result, the researchers concluded that sildenafil could be a more effective treatment for erectile dysfunction (ED) than angina and switched the focus of their studies to develop a medication to treat erectile dysfunction in men.

Accordingly, sildenafil went through clinical trials in the early 1990s, received a patent in 1996, and gained FDA approval in the US. In 1998, Pfizer launched sildenafil under the brand name Viagra to treat erectile dysfunction in the US and worldwide, generating peak annual sales in this indication of over $2 billion.

Pfizer continued to study sildenafil's potentially therapeutic effects of inhibiting PDE5 and proposed exploiting the vasodilation properties it produces to treat pulmonary arterial hypertension at one-fifth of the dose used in erectile dysfunction.

Considered a rare disease (2 to 3 million cases per year), the idiopathic form of pulmonary hypertension is fatal. Pfizer realized this opportunity by repositioning sildenafil under a new brand name, Revatio®, for a second time to treat pulmonary arterial hypertension(PAH). The rare disease status of the condition made it easy for Pfizer to obtain approval for a second sildenafil product (Revatio®) in 2005 in this new condition.

Source: Adapted from articles—1. Jean-Pierre Jourdan, Ronan Bureau, Christophe Rochais, Patrick Dailemagne, *Drug Repositioning: A Brief Overview*, Journal of Pharmacy and Pharmacology / Volume 72, Issue 9, p. 1145—1151, Wiley Online Library, 2. Medically Reviewed by Kristin Hall, FNP, Written by Editorial Team at HIMS (Health Management Information System), Revatio Vs. Viagra: What's the Difference? HIMS, September 2, 2020)

CASE

45

Repositioned Drugs Making A Beeline for Alzheimer's Drug Treatment!

Alzheimer's disease is one for which no new drugs have been marketed since galantamine in 2000. That is why so many drug repositioning trials are being conducted in this field, albeit unsuccessfully. In 2017, over 100 drugs were undergoing clinical trials for Alzheimer's Disease.

About twenty-seven of these drugs have already been marketed and are therefore being investigated for repositioning. The following table lists the previously approved drugs undergoing clinical trials in Alzheimer's Disease.

Table 3.3 List of Repositioning Drugs in Development For Alzheimer's Disease

Molecule	Mechanism of Action	Original Indication
Aripiprazole	Dopaminergic Agonist	Atypical Antipsychotic
Brexipiprazole	Dopaminergic Agonist	Atypical Antipsychotic
Insulin	Insulin Receptor Ligand	Types 1 and 2 Diabetes
Methylphenidate	Dopamine Reuptake Inhibitor	ADHD
Nabilone	Cannabinoid	Nausea, Vomiting
Nilvadipine	Calcium Channel Antagonist, Dihydropyridines	Prinzmetal's angina, Hypertension, Raynaud's phenomenon
Pioglitazone	PPARγ Agonist Receptor	Type 2 Diabetes
Atomoxetine	Adrenaline Reuptake Inhibitor	ADHD
Candesartran	Angiotensin Agonist Receptor	Hypertension

Table 3.3 *Contd...*

Molecule	Mechanism of Action	Original Indication
Cilostazol	PDE3 Inhibitor	Intermittent Claudication
Dronabinol	Cannabinoid	Nausea, Vomiting
Formoterol	B-2 Adrenergic Receptor Agonist	Asthma
Detemir Insulin	Insulin Receptor Ligand	Types 1 and 2 Diabetes
Glulisine Insulin	Insulin Receptor Ligand	Types 1 and 2 Diabetes

(Source: Jean-Pierre Jourdan, Ronan Bureau, Christophe Rochais, Patrick Dailemagne, Drug Repositioning: A Brief Overview, Journal of Pharmacy and Pharmacology / Volume 72, Issue 9, 9. 1145-1154, Wiley Online Library).

The high proportion of existing drugs in the Alzheimer's disease pipeline indicates the increasing reliance on repositioning.

(Source: 1. Jean-Pierre Jourdan, Ronan Bureau, Christophe Rochais, Patrick Dailemagne, *Drug Repositioning: A Brief Overview*, Journal of Pharmacy and Pharmacology / Volume 72, Issue 9, p. 1145—1151, Wiley Online Library)

CASE

46

Antihypertensive Minoxidil Gets Repurposed To Treat Baldness!

In the late 1950s, Upjohn (Pfizer, now), a global pharmaceutical company, developed minoxidil as a treatment for ulcers, but to the scientist's disappointment, the drug did not cure ulcers. However, they were pleasantly surprised to observe that minoxidil showed a vasodilation effect. So the company further developed minoxidil tablets to treat hypertension and obtained US FDA approval for treating high blood pressure in 1979.

When patients taking the antihypertensive agent minoxidil in clinical trials in the late 1960s started getting a bit hairy, executives at Upjohn— the US pharmaceutical company that made the drug, initially dismissed it as a harmless side effect but soon realized that it could be a great opportunity, and repurposed it to develop minoxidil liquid that can be applied to the scalp directly for hair growth.

By the 1980s, doctors were widely prescribing minoxidil to their balding patients off-label. Finally, in 1988, the FDA approved minoxidil as a treatment for baldness in men under the brand name, Rogaine®. FDA rejected the brand name of Upjohn's first choice, Regain, as misleading.

In 1991, Upjohn made the product available for women. Later in February 1996, FDA approved both the over-the-counter sale of Rogaine® and generic formulations as minoxidil's patent expired.

(Source: The Accidental Discovery of Minoxidil and Other Medicines, Hims, **forhims.com**)

CHAPTER

4

Blue Ocean Strategy

Blue Ocean strategists do not seek to beat the competition. Instead, they aim to make competition irrelevant.

— W. Chan Kim, Professor of Strategy and Management at INSEAD Business School in France and Co-Author of the book, Blue Ocean Strategy

Blue and Red Oceans

W. Chan Kim and Renée Mauborgne used blue and red oceans as a metaphor for describing the market universe in their highly acclaimed book, *Blue Ocean Strategy*. Red Oceans are all industries in existence today – the known marketplace. In Red Oceans, industry boundaries are defined and accepted, and the competitive rules of the game are known. In the Red Ocean market space companies try to outperform their rivals, and grab a more significant share of the product, or market demand. The prospects for profits and growth are reduced in red oceans as the market space gets crowded. Cutthroat competition turns red oceans bloody hence the metaphorical name red oceans.

Blue Oceans, on the contrary, denotes all the industries that are not in existence today – the unknown market space untainted by competition. Blue Oceans provide ample opportunities for rapid growth and profits as there is no competition. Competition is irrelevant as the rules for the game are waiting to be set. Blue Ocean is an analogy to describe market space's wider, deeper potential that is not yet explored. The following table presents the key differences between Red Ocean and Blue Ocean market spaces at a glance:

Table 4.1 Red and Blue Oceans: Key Differences

Red Ocean Strategies	Blue Ocean Strategies
1. Competing in existing market space.	Create uncontested market space.
2. Beat the competition.	Make the competition irrelevant.
3. Make the value / cost tradeoff.	Break the value / cost tradeoff.
4. Align the whole system of a company's activities with strategic choice of differentiation or low cost.	Align the whole system of a company's activities in the pursuit of differentiation and low cost.

(Source: Blue Ocean Strategy, Harvard Business Review, October 2004)

Value Innovation

The bedrock of the blue ocean strategy is value innovation. What is value innovation? Value innovation is creating value simultaneously for both the buyer and the company. Charles W. L. Hill, a Michigan State University professor, first proposed the value innovation concept. He claimed that Porter's Five Forces Framework for competitive analysis was inadequate because differentiation can be a means to achieve low cost. Instead, he suggested combining differentiation and low cost may be necessary for firms to achieve sustainable competitive advantage. The core idea of a blue ocean strategy is to create a leap in value for both— the company and its sellers by breaking a tradeoff between differentiation and low cost.

Later in 2004, W. Chan Kim and Renée Mauborgne, professors at INSEAD business school in France, came out with the Blue Ocean Strategy that explains the what, why, and how of creating Blue Ocean strategies in today's predominantly Red-Ocean marketplace. The core idea here, too, is based on value innovation. Value innovation is creating value simultaneously for both, the buyer and the company. You create a Blue Ocean when you raise the market's value (in product, service, or delivery) while simultaneously reducing or eliminating features or functions that are less valued by the current or future market (customers). The essence of value innovation is best captured in the statement of Akio Morita, Chairman of Sony Corporation, when he pioneered the concept of value innovation in the personal music industry with the introduction of the Walkman:

Carefully watch how people live, get an intuitive sense of what they might want, and then go with it. Don't do market research.

This careful observation created a new, uncontested market space in 1979 with the introduction of the Walkman. Henry Ford's Model-T Car offers another classic example of how the value of innovation created a blue ocean in the automobile industry at the time. W. Chan Kim and Renée Mauborgne clearly explain how Henry Ford used the value innovation to create an uncontested market space for his Model-T Car, in their Harvard Business Review Article of October 2004, on *Blue Ocean Strategy*:

CASE

47

Henry Ford Creates A Blue Ocean!

The automobile industry was small and unattractive at the end of the 19th century. It was crammed with over 500 automakers competing in the crowded market for handmade luxury cars. The average price of the car was around US $1,500. Only the very rich could afford it. The industry, as a result, was so unpopular that it led to even an anti-car activist movement. The anti-car activists tore up roads, ringed parked cars with barbed wire, and organized boycotts of car-driving business people and politicians to demonstrate their protests.

Henry Ford did not want to swim in this Red Ocean. So, instead of trying to beat the competition for a slice of the share in this heavily contested market, he reconstructed the industry boundaries of cars and horse-drawn carriages, competing in the same space as local transportation. Horse-drawn carriages were the primary means of local transportation across America. The major advantage of the horse-drawn carriages over automobiles was that they could easily negotiate the bumps and dirt roads that were everywhere in America, which the automobiles at the time could not.

Henry Ford understood the market situation enough to break away from the competition and unlock the enormous untapped potential demand. He built Model-T Car and called it *for the multitude (not only for the rich) constructed with the best materials*. Ford built a car as the horse-drawn carriage meant for everyday use. Model-T car came in just one color, black, and there were a few optional extras. It was durable, reliable, and designed to travel effortlessly on dirt roads in rain, snow, or sunshine. People could learn to drive it easily.

The pricing strategy, too, was different. Ford did not look at the automobile industry for a price point; he looked at the horse-drawn carriages, which cost $400 on average. In 1908, the first Model T cost $850. In 1909, the price dropped to $609, and by 1924, it was down to $290. The mass production with its pioneering assembly line operation of Model-T car made the price drops possible.

Ford Motor Company transformed the industry boundaries, achieved value innovation, created an uncontested market space, and made the competition irrelevant. Ford created a Blue Ocean!

(Source: Blue Ocean Strategy, Harvard Business Review, October 2004)

How to Formulate a Blue Ocean Strategy?

Understand that Blue Ocean is a journey and not a destination. It challenges everything you thought you knew about strategic success in the marketplace. It provides a systematic approach to making the competition irrelevant. To formulate a Blue Ocean strategy, you must take a critical look at yourself, your business, and your path. The 'Pioneer - Migrator - Settler Map' (PMS Map) can help you as a diagnostic tool to start taking stock of where your products and services fit into your industry.

The PMS Map

The Pioneer - Migrator - Settler Map is a diagnostic tool that shows how your revenue-generating products and services contribute to the company's future growth. The map helps you to determine if you are in the Red Ocean, fighting for your life, or enjoying the tranquility of the deep blue waters of the Blue Ocean where there is no competition in sight. You can organize the key products into three categories and display them by size even. Once you analyze and understand the current positions of your products and services regarding their relative positions on the PMS Map, you can move them to the more desirable stages from where they are now. Here is a brief description of what these labels - Pioneer, Migrator, and Settler stand for:

1. The **Pioneers** are products that offer unprecedented value with high-profit growth potential. They are unique products and virtually free from competition. They have the entire market for themselves.
2. The **Migrators** are products with exceptional value but not innovative, and these products sit on the boundaries of the Red and Blue oceans. They may offer some value and potential for profit growth if you make some changes.
3. The **Settlers** are products that follow the industry norms with little or no differentiation. They are not innovative and not much different from the competition and, therefore, do not offer much potential for profit growth. Also, these products face a shrinking customer pool. Settlers are primarily in the Red Ocean space.

The PMS Map

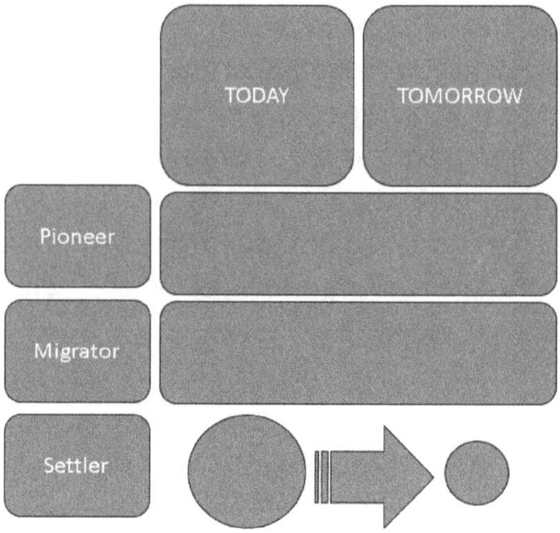

Figure 4.1 The PMS Map

Blue Ocean Strategy: Key Questions

Blue Ocean Strategy is a shift in mindset. You need to expand your mental horizons and shift your understanding to find out where the opportunity lies. You need to ask a fundamentally different set of questions. The answers to such questions would then enable you to perceive the fallacies and limitations of long-held beliefs and conventional thinking and the consequent boundaries we impose on ourselves. Here are the necessary steps involved in migrating your products which are currently settlers (swimming in the bloody Red Ocean) to the status of pioneers (enjoying the tranquility of the vast, deep Blue Ocean space with no competition in sight):

1. Get a clear idea about the current state of play in your industry.
2. Find out and uncover the hidden pain points that limit the industry's current size and discover an ocean of non-customers.
3. Find out how to reconstruct your market boundaries and explore blue ocean opportunities.
4. Select the right Blue Ocean to move, conduct a rapid market test, and launch.

Identifying Non-Customers

Last but not least is the identification of non-customers. It is the most crucial step in implementing a Blue Ocean Strategy. In Red Oceans, the competition leads to a shrinking pool of customers for whose attention all the players are fighting. Such competition naturally leads to erosion of profit margins. Instead, if you can find a market (a large pool of customers) within the boundaries of our existing target market — one that has not been reached— we can open up a new market where there is no competition. W. Chan Kim and Renée Mauborgne suggest in their Blue Ocean Strategy three tiers of non-customers:

1. The first tier consists of existing customers looking to leave the industry. We need to find out the pain points responsible for this decision.
2. The second tier consists of those who consciously decide against your product or service. What are customers looking for? What should we do to meet their latent needs and remove their pain points in our current offering?
3. The third tier contains people who are in distant markets. What are the key differences between our existing markets and those distant markets? How can we transform the boundaries of both — our current markets and those distant markets?

Eventually, Blue Oceans turn red when more players enter their space. The companies must, therefore, continuously explore to find the Blue Ocean opportunities or uncontested market spaces to stay at the top of the market. Pharmaceutical markets are Red Ocean markets. The industry offers its Blue Ocean periods for those companies who can create uncontested spaces every time they are at their innovative best. Successful pharmaceutical companies continually explore the market space to create their Blue Ocean strategies.

The following four cases show how some of the world's leading pharmaceutical companies have created uncontested market spaces with their Blue Ocean strategies for their products and reaped rich dividends.

CASE

48

Novo Nordisk's Blue Ocean Strategy!

How do you create a blue ocean strategy? By challenging the conventional wisdom in any given industry. By challenging the prevailing mental model. By rediscovering the market needs in markets that are mature and saturated. By shifting the way of looking at customer needs from the functional to the emotional. Companies that look at various customer groups can gain new insights into designing their value proposition to focus on previously overlooked customer needs.

That is what exactly Novo Nordisk had done with its Novopen. Novo Nordisk, the Danish insulin producer, broke away from the competition and created a blue ocean by shifting the industry's longstanding focus on doctors to the users — patients themselves.

Diabetic patients use insulin to regulate their blood sugar levels. Historically, the insulin industry, like the pharmaceutical industry, focused on the key influencers: doctors. However, it is the doctors who prescribe insulin to their patients. Therefore, the industry sharpened its Attention and efforts to produce purer insulin in response to doctors' quest for better medication. The innovations in purification technology had improved dramatically in the 1980s, and there was minimal scope to develop it further. Novo Nordisk, the leader in the insulin industry, had already created the first human monocomponent insulin that was chemically the exact copy of human insulin. The competition was rapidly catching on.

Novo Nordisk saw that it could break away from the competition and create a new market by shifting the industry's longstanding focus on doctors to the users. In focusing on patients, Novo Nordisk found that most diabetic patients were uncomfortable using syringes to administer insulin injections. Considering a diabetic needs to inject himself three or four times a day, using the syringe is daunting. Moreover, there was a social stigma attached to using a needle and vial in public. Novo Nordisk thus broke through a prevailing mental model by shifting from a functional to an emotional (and social) need. As a result, it led to the creation of the Novopen, a patient-friendly drug delivery device for people with diabetes. Rajiv Narang and Devika Devaiah narrate this exciting story of how exactly this had happened in their book, *Orbit-shifting Innovations: The dynamics of ideas that created history*:

In January 1981, Sonnich Fryland, the marketing director of Novo Nordisk, called John. Rex, the head of packaging, and Ivan Jensen, a doctor, into his room. Fryland removed his fountain pen from his pocket and asked whether it would be possible to produce a device that looked like a fountain pen that could hold a week's supply of insulin and administer two units of insulin at the touch of a button. Of course, the pen had to be simple and discreet and look like an actual fountain pen.

That is how Novo Nordisk seized the blue ocean opportunity of *Novopen*, launched in 1985. *Novopen* is the first user-friendly insulin delivery solution designed to remove the hassle and embarrassment of administering insulin. The *Novopen* resembled a fountain pen; it contained an insulin cartridge that allowed the patient to comfortably carry roughly a week's insulin requirement in one self-contained unit. In addition, the pen had an integrated click mechanism, making it possible even for blind patients to control the dosing and administer insulin.

Novo Nordisk continued to dominate the blue ocean it had unlocked. The company pursued a continuous innovation program. Introduced in 1989, *Novolet* is a pre-filled disposable insulin injection pen with a dosing system that provides users with even greater convenience and ease of use. In 1999, the company introduced *Innovo*, integrated electronic memory and cartridge-based delivery system. *Innovo* was designed to manage insulin delivery through built-in memory and display the dose, the last dose, and the elapsed time — information critical for reducing risk and eliminating worries about missing a dose.

Thus, Novo Nordisk shifted the industry landscape and transformed the company from an insulin manufacturing and marketing company to a diabetes care company. The company had always been a dominant player in the insulin market. The difference today is that about 70 percent of the company's total turnover comes from diabetes care, which originated mostly in the company's thinking regarding users rather than influencers. In other words, from the Blue Ocean that it had created.

(Source: Adapted from Rajiv Narang and Devika Devaiah's book, *Orbit-shifting Innovations: The dynamics of ideas that created history*)

CASE

49

The Little Blue Pill's Astonishing Dream Run!

Viagra, launched in America twenty years ago, is today's most ubiquitous pharmaceutical brand name. Type it into Google, and a search throws up more than four million references; ten times more than Prozac and 20 times as many as Botox, its nearest competitors.

Indeed, the takeoff of Viagra was one of the fastest that a new drug has ever seen. Almost immediately after its launch in the United States, it was being prescribed at 10,000 a day. It was unprecedented for a prescription drug. In Atlanta, urologist Dr. John Stripling reportedly wrote about 300 prescriptions on the day Viagra was available.

Accidental Discovery

For all the great success that Viagra achieved, its discovery was accidental and not a result of focused research. Two British scientists— Peter Dunn and Albert Wood at Pfizer, created sildenafil citrate, a new chemical entity (NCE). They believed that the drug would be useful in treating high blood pressure and angina. However, as they were employees of Pfizer at the time, they were not allowed to discuss the status of the invention.

In 1994, Dr. Nicholas Terret and his colleague Peter Ellis found that sildenafil can enhance blood flow to the penile region in patients with erectile dysfunction. In addition, they discovered that sildenafil increases the relaxing muscle effects of nitric oxide, a chemical released during sexual stimulation. This relaxation of the muscle in the penis allows a higher blood flow rate and aids in producing an erection. Dr. Nicholas Terret was named in the British patent for sildenafil citrate.

Pfizer completed several trials of sildenafil citrate, but none provided any hope of treating heart diseases. However, Ian Osterloh, a researcher, observed an interesting side effect of the drug during the trials. Volunteers of the trail were reporting increased erections several days after taking the drug. An interesting coincidence was that around the same time, other studies were revealing more information about the biochemical pathways involved in the erection process. It helped the Pfizer team of scientists to understand how the drug might amplify the process of erection. Dr. Simon Campbell, a Pfizer veteran, submitted a research proposal for further investigation and handed over the project to another research team. Although Dr. Simon Campbell did not invent sildenafil citrate, which later became Viagra, he is called the father of Viagra because he laid the seed and started the project. He was later Knighted. Viagra indeed was a serendipitous discovery!

Viagra in the Media

Thousands of stories were written in the popular press about Viagra between September 1996 and the product's eventual launch in late March 1998. No other prescription drug brand received as much media attention as Viagra did. Jay Baglia, Assistant Professor in the department of communication studies at San Jose University at the time, describes in his well-researched book, *The Viagra AdVenture*, four phases of media coverage from September 1996 to October 2002. Viagra was frequently introduced in these articles through the use of emphatic epithets. Here are some of the more important ones:

- Eighteen months before its launch, Viagra was characterized as the *Ultimate erection aid* in a Newsweek article by Geoffrey

Cowley titled, *Attention: Aging Men*.

- The New York Times called Viagra, *A Wonder of the Modern Age*; *The New Miracle Drug* and; *The New National Drug of Choice*.
- Newsweek followed its earlier article with *The Potency Wonder Drug.*
- The US News & World Report called Viagra, *The Sexual Potency Drug*.

All these monickers imply that this technology is something we have all been waiting for. Also, Douglas Martin's article in the New York Times, *Thanks a Bunch Viagra: The Pill that Revived Sex, or At Least Talking About It*, suggested that Viagra's availability got people talking about sex generally, and got men to visit their doctors. After generations of taboo refusing to talk about sexual failure, erectile dysfunction has become a subject that one can discuss openly. Erica Jung, the author, summed up best this great transformation that media had brought about when she said: *Impotence was the great secret. Now, suddenly, you can't go to a dinner party without people talking about erections!*

Marketing Excellence

Viagra is a classic example of marketing excellence in action. Pfizer's first strategic masterstroke was its embarkation on the rebranding of impotence itself. Impotence suggested a lack of power, a referendum on a man's masculinity and humanity. Instead of talking about impotence, Pfizer chose to speak of Viagra regarding male enhancement. It adopted the medicalized language of erectile dysfunction and offered a straightforward and convenient medical solution. Furthermore, the company made the condition look like a common condition through its marketing communication — that half of men over 40 are affected with 'ED.' How can something so common be shameful?

The second brilliant marketing move was to hire Bob Dole, a former presidential nominee, a war veteran, and an elder statesman, as Viagra's spokesman. With this, Pfizer brought a gendered notion of power and patriotism to Viagra marketing and made the sexual function a metaphor for masculine dignity. Bob Dole appeared on a Larry King Live Show in 1998 to discuss his struggles with erectile dysfunction and his battle with prostate cancer. He even talked about the effect the battle had on his body even after the battle was won — and told the viewers about the medical solution he had found for the disorder. The company later used Bob Dole in a TV ad that instantly became iconic. Dole, however, did not talk about Viagra itself in the ad. The little blue pill in all this talk of heroism was merely implied.

Pfizer's third winning move in its marketing was that it successfully attempted to reclaim the notions of potency from the ideas of impotence, which it had almost antiquated. The company recruited celebrities from the sports world, such as NASCAR driver Mark Martin, the soccer legend Pele, and the baseball player Rafael Palmer to star in ads to accomplish this. The ads featuring these sports celebrities emphasized men being classically manly: speeding, winning, overcoming. The taglines used for these ads were: *Love life again and Step up to the plate*. The ads always signed off with an - Ask your doctor.

Viagra Advertising

How did Pfizer develop such great ads that resonated with its target audience? Pfizer followed the same principles and procedures it would follow for its drug discovery program. To unearth an ad or a TV commercial that would resonate with its audience, it developed a screening system that would parallel its drug discovery program. Pfizer's vice president for consumer marketing, Dorothy Wetzel, explained: *Just as the Pfizer research and development screened thousands of different components to find the one that makes a difference, we are trying to apply the same process to our communication development; getting multiple agencies to develop ideas and screen it down to the one killer communication.*

After relying on metaphorical ads featuring older men using horses to get their trucks out of mud, or figuring out how to get the factory works unclogged, Viagra tried a more direct and bold approach: having a woman encourage men to get treatment for erectile dysfunction. The new TV ad spot from BBDO shows a forty-something woman with a British accent and slinky dress, saying:

You know what, plenty of guys have this issue...If ED is stopping what you started, ask your doctor about Viagra...

This ad is almost an endorsement from the women of Viagra.

The competition for erectile dysfunction scripts was heating up if ad spends of 2014 were any indication. Two erectile dysfunction drugs were among the top ten in ad spending. Eli Lilly took the top spot for ad spend in 2014. It was the number one spender with $272 million, followed by Viagra at number four with an ad spend of $232 million.

With US sales of $1.14 billion and worldwide sales of over $2 billion in 2016, after eighteen years since its approval, Viagra had a dream run! The following table presents a timeline of Viagra's dream run.

Table 4.1 Viagra's Dream Run: A Timeline

Timeline	Activity
1989	Prizer scientists in Great Britain, Peter Dunn and Albert Wood created a drug called sildenafil citrate that they believed would be useful in treating high blood pressure and angina.
1990s (Early)	Sildenafil showed little or no hope of treating high blood pressure and angina in the trials. However, an interesting side effect was observed during the clinical trials. The volunteers in the trials reported increased erections several days after taking the drug.
1991	Dr. Nicholas Terret is named in the British patent for sildenafil citrate (Trade name Viagra) as a heart medication. Terret is often considered as the father of Viagra.
1996	Pfizer patents sildenafil in the United States.

Table 4.1 *Contd...*

Timeline	Activity
March 1998	The US FDA approves Viagra for treating erectile dysfunction. In the following weeks, US pharmacists dispense more than 40,000 prescriptions.
May 1998	Viagra gets unprecedented media attention: A. Time magazine's cover story quotes the Penthouse publisher Bob Guccione as saying: *We believe Viagra will free the American male Libido.* B. On CNN's Larry King Live show, former presidential nominee, Bob Dole admits that he took part in experimental trials of Viagra calling it a great drug.
June 1998	Newsweek calls Viagra *the hottest new drug in history — almost anywhere in the world.* At the time Viagra was being marketed only in the United States, Mexico, Brazil and Morocco, but Newsweek reports growing black market sales in other countries.
December 1998	A. Pfizer hires Bob Dole, a former Presidential nominee for a television campaign aimed at raising awareness of male impotence. B. The Washington Post reports that CIA was using Viagra to gain friends in Afghanistan. While CIA had a long history of buying information with cash, the growing insurgency had prompted the use of novel incentives and creative bargaining to get information.
July 1999	Popular TV show, *Sex and the City* airs *The Man, The Myth, and Viagra* in which, character Samatha dates a wealthy Alderman, who uses the *little blue pills.* In the next season, Samantha takes the *little blue pills* herself to enhance her sexual experiences.
2000	Dr. Sanjay Kaul presents research at the 49th Annual Scientific Session of American College of Cardiology that suggests 522 patients died while taking Viagra in the first year the drug was on the market. However, there was no implication of cause-and-effect relationship.
August 2003	The US FDA approves Bayer Corporation's vardenafil hydrochloride (Levitra) to treat erectile dysfunction.
November 2003	The US FDA approves Lilly Icos' tadalafil (Cialis) to treat erectile dysfunction.
2011	A Federal Judge extends Pfizer's US patent for Viagra, making sure that generic versions of Viagra cannot come to market until 2020.

Table 4.1 *Contd...*

Timeline	Activity
April 2012	The US FDA approves a new erectile dysfunction drug called avanafil, which will be sold under the brand name of Stendra. Stendra, which is taken as-needed basis 30 minutes before the sexual activity is a product of Vivus, a small pharmaceutical company headquartered in Campbell, California.
2013	A. Cialis of Eli Lilly overtakes Viagra for the first time in global sales. B. Teva settles a Viagra patent litigation with Pfizer and enters into an agreement to market generic version of Viagra from December 2017.
2014	Viagra plans ahead and gets ready to face the impending genericization in 2020: A. Introduces a *singles* pack B. Launches a massive DTC campaign Goes on line for selling Viagra as a prescription drug, which is first for a Big Pharma company
2015	Mylan settles a patent litigation related to Viagra with Pfizer and gets ready to launch generic Viagra in the US in December 2017.
2017	Pfizer gets Pharmacy (P) approval for its Viagra Connect 50 mg film-coated tablets by MHRA in the United Kingdom in November 2017. Pfizer can market Viagra Connect directly to consumers through pharmacists without prescriptions.

Pfizer Gets Ready for Viagra's Genericization

Competition for Viagra was heating up with new entrants such as Levitra (co-marketed by Bayer and GlaxoSmithKline in the US) and Cialis (Eli Lilly). The Viagra patents, too, were nearing their expiries in some markets. The drug makers were flooding television, radio, magazines, newspapers, and even mailboxes with their advertising messages. The drug makers were sponsoring sports like golf and auto racing. Levitra and Cialis had even tried Super Bowl advertising. They paid more than $4 million each for 60-second commercial spots during the game in February 2012. Finally, Cialis had overtaken Pfizer as the market leader with world sales of $1.9 billion at the end of 2012. Pfizer had been actively planning to counter competition and protect its market share from the impending generic erosion. Some of the more important moves that Pfizer undertook were:

1. Launching a generic version of Viagra in New Zealand under a different brand name— Avigra, in 2011. Avigra was made available in New Zealand at a competitive price to those men who want to remain on it. Avigra, the second brand of Pfizer's Viagra, retails for about half the price of Viagra Classic. The price was more than other generics, but the discount was significant enough to tempt consumers, who are sensitive to price.
2. Pfizer attempted to rethink the typical drug starter pack of three tablets in a box. That was almost the industry practice. Instead, it drew inspiration from Z-Pack (5 tablets in a box) and departed from the norm. Why this change? The Viagra team recognized the importance of the first experience for all people suffering from ED. They knew that clinically, it might take a few tries for the people to get the drug's full effect. To ensure that the people with ED should get the full effect with the first starter pack, they increased the number of tablets.
3. Publication of *Voices*, a custom publication service of Viagra for the waiting rooms at doctors' offices in the United States to improve awareness and knowledge about the condition, ED. *Voices* covered important personalities from sports, entertainment, and members of Earth, Wind & Fire - weighing in on the importance of taking charge of their health. *Voices* also attempted to dispel the myths surrounding erectile dysfunction. Men could pick up *Voices* in the doctors' offices, and the other patients would not necessarily recognize it as a Viagra piece.
4. Introduction of chewable form Viagra in Mexico in 2012, before its patent expiry under the brand name Viagra Jet.
5. Introduction of Viagra in single packs to help men with erectile dysfunction treat their condition when needed. Pfizer conducted an online survey of 200 men, and 16 percent of them reported that they were taking Viagra outside the home. The company introduced the single packs to refresh an aging brand, making purchasing more convenient.

6. Entering into an agreement with two leading international generic manufacturers, Teva and Mylan, in the US to bring out their respective generic versions by the end of 2017. Teva and Mylan would pay a certain amount as royalty on the sales of their generic versions under the agreement.
7. Selling of Viagra, the prescription drug online began in 2012. In a first for the drug industry, Pfizer decided to make Viagra available online. Patients still needed a prescription to buy Viagra online but no longer had to face a pharmacist to get the drug. Pfizer offered three free pills with the first order, and a 30 percent discount on the second order. This bold move blew up the drug industry's distribution model. Pharmaceutical companies do not sell their products directly to patients. Instead, they sell their products in bulk to wholesalers, who then distribute them to pharmacists, hospitals, and doctors' offices.
8. Launching an OTC version of Viagra in the United Kingdom under the brand name Viagra Connect.
9. Introduction of a frequent user Value Card offering a free seventh prescription from each six customer refills.
10. Introduction of mobile texting for Viagra discounts. In what seemed to be the first for a pharmaceutical company, Pfizer's new TV commercial of 2017 for Viagra encouraged patients to text a keyword from their mobile phones to receive special discounts. The ad opened with the now familiar woman in a dark blue dress, who asked: *Guys, want to save 50 percent on a year-long supply of Viagra for ED?* A mobile phone close-up takes over the screen with the promotion and text keyword "VSAVE," and she explains how to get the discount in voiceover.

Viagra Connect

Pfizer got Pharmacy (P) approval in November 2017, to market its 50 mg film-coated sildenafil tablets by the Medicines and Healthcare Regulatory Authority (MHRA) in the United Kingdom. These tablets were to be sold under the brand name; *Viagra Connect* through pharmacists directly to the consumers without a prescription. Pharmacy (P) is an over-the-counter approval where pharmacists can dispense medicines without prescriptions in the UK. *Viagra Connect* retailed for £19.99 for a four-tablet pack, and £34.99 for eight tablets. The reclassification of *Viagra Connect* from prescription-only medicine (POM) to pharmacy (P) status increased safe access to sildenafil. In addition, it ensured that patients got good, accurate advice if it was right for them.

Viagra Connect went on sale in the UK in the third week of April 2018, and was available in pharmacies without prescriptions, unlike standard Viagra medication.

To support the launch of Viagra Connect, Pfizer unveiled extensive training for the product to pharmacists on March 12, 2018. This largest-ever program for pharmacists includes e-learning modules, face-to-face sessions, and regional meetings. In addition, Pfizer provided all the participating pharmacists with tips on managing conversations. It is important because pharmacists need to become familiar with the indications and contraindications and how to counsel those seeking sildenafil, as conversations may involve teasing out some sensitive information.

Digital training available to the participants included videos, interactive content, and print-and-keep resources. The site also included a *Viagra Connect* Checklist. Tailored content was also available to pharmacy assistants, who may be the first point of contact for men presenting to the pharmacy with erectile dysfunction symptoms.

The training was free of charge for pharmacists and pharmacy staff, including access to 23 regional training events with two places allocated per pharmacy on a first-come-first-serve basis.

The Viagra Connect DTC Campaign

Pfizer launched a new direct-to-consumer (DTC) campaign to overturn the stigma surrounding erectile dysfunction and increase patient traffic for its new over-the-counter *Viagra Connect* to the pharmacies in the UK. These ads were created by Tony Malcolm, Josh Pearce, and Sean Johnson at Y & R (Young & Rubicam), London. This ad campaign aims to raise awareness of erectile dysfunction in the UK and communicate the normality of the condition among men. In addition, the copy of ads creatively delivers the message that erectile dysfunction is a common condition that can be treated without needing a prescription. There were three ads released, and the copy of each ad is presented below:

Copy of the Sport-focused Ad

4.3 Million men in the UK experience erectile problems. That's a lot of men. That's enough men to fill every major British football stadium. That's more men than people who went to a rugby match last year. That's more men than everyone who goes to the gym every day. So a lot of men will be glad to know that Viagra Connect is now Available without a prescription.

viagraconnect.co.uk Viagra Connect

Copy of the Travel-Focused Ad

4.3 Million men in the UK experience erectile problems. That's a lot of men. That's 49,000 buses worth, in fact. That is more men there than are cabs in the whole of the UK. That's more men than there are cars in London. More men than people who cycled to work yesterday. More men than people who will use the tube today. More men than all the red buses in the world. More men than there are flights out-of-the UK in a whole year, even. So a lot of men will be glad to know that Viagra Connect is now available without a prescription.

viagraconnect.co.uk Viagra Connect

Copy of the News-focused Ad

4.3 Million men in the UK Experience erectile problems. That's a lot of men. That's more men than there are words in this newspaper. In fact, that's twenty-five times more Men than there are words in the English language. More men than all the words in all the novels of Charles Dickens ever wrote, even. So many men will be glad to know that Viagra Connect is available without a prescription.

viagraconnect.co.uk Viagra Connect

These ads have used very creatively the incredibly large number of 4.3 million to communicate compellingly how common erectile dysfunction is, and that help is available just for the asking. It was the first phase of the creative campaign, and more ads would follow. A media strategy supported by Wavemaker includes social and content partnerships, and public relations (PR) activity by Burson Cohn & Wolfe.

Success Beyond Compare

You cannot view the success of Viagra in financial terms alone. It had been a phenomenal success, no doubt, but there is more to Viagra's success than meets the eye. Than just sales and profits alone. Viagra did make sales and profits, plenty of them. In fact, Viagra became a darling of Wall Street. After introducing Viagra in 1998, Pfizer became the fifth most profitable corporation in the world by 2002. Such was the commercial success of Viagra. However, then, there is more to Viagra.

Lynne Luciano, in her book, *Looking Good: Male Body Image in Modern America*, writes of ED as a circular malady:

The more it was talked about, the more of it there was. Something similar had happened with Viagra— while it arrived on the market at the tail end of the 1990s, it eclipsed both Penicillin and the Birth control pill to become the most talked about drug of the century!

Viagra, the brand name drug as we know it, may no longer be the market force it once was. However, even then, there is no question that its impact on two decades of conversations about modern sex and the de-stigmatization of erectile dysfunction has been incredible.

Finally, what can you say about Viagra, and how do you explain its phenomenal success? As Jamie Reidy, an early salesman of Pfizer's game-changing drug, in his book, The Hard Sell: The evolution of a Viagra salesman, says: *This isn't a pill. It's a revolution!*

Lessons

The marketing of Viagra offers many valuable lessons for pharmaceutical marketers. Firstly, It provides a blueprint for medicalizing a lifestyle condition — impotence, that was almost considered taboo to discuss in public and was embarrassing to talk about even with physicians. Pfizer changed it with its marketing, advertising, and public relations strategies. Lisa Stockman of Inventiv health put it succinctly when she said: *No matter what anybody said or did, Impotence had little chance of being thought of as a medical condition. Erectile Dysfunction did.*

Pfizer's brand and marketing teams realized that the current perception of impotence could limit the drug's impact on the lives of the needy patients, and the bottom line. The solution was to launch a focused educational effort before the launch of Viagra. The result? Pfizer's educational effort went down in pharmaceutical marketing history as the first and most effective medicalization campaign.

It was not an easy task. First, Pfizer had to give the reluctant physicians a reason to have a conversation about the condition. That meant linking erectile dysfunction to the things familiar to physicians and the things they were traditionally concerned about, such as diseases like diabetes and cardiac problems. So the conversation started something like this: *Doctor, you should be asking about ED because it often happens eighteen months before a cardiac event.*

Pfizer followed the same approach even for its media campaigns. The company subtly explained and tried to show the impact of ED on men, regarding emotional well-being and depression, beyond the effect on sex lives.

Secondly, Pfizer showed a way to create a therapeutic category. Impotence was thoroughly stigmatized as both a condition and a word. By recasting impotence as erectile dysfunction, Pfizer could dodge the toxic attitudinal predisposition towards the condition.

Thirdly, Pfizer showed the industry how to get the best out of DTCA campaigns for Viagra. Pfizer was not the first to use a celebrity endorsement for its disease awareness campaigns. However, it ushered in the era of the celebrity spokesperson. When the long-term senator, former presidential candidate, and an honored war veteran, Bob Dole, appeared in a Viagra commercial in 1998, he revolutionized the way such personalities participated in pharmaceutical campaigns. It had encouraged pharmaceutical companies to aim higher in their pursuit of celebrity endorsers and advocates. Here is a message Bob Dole delivered in a TV commercial that resonated with its target audience: *It is a little embarrassing to talk about ED, but it's so important to millions of men and their partners that I decided to talk about it publicly.*

Fourth, Viagra's media strategy shows us how to obliterate the media's reluctance to cover embarrassing health-related stories. Pfizer's media and public relations teams sat down with physicians and scientists and spent much time before the launch. Their counsel mainly helped in underpinning the medical and psychological impact of ED. As a result, the media that was once reluctant to do any story on impotence made an about turn to push Viagra into pop culture and the family living room conversation. As a result, a record two-billion impressions within a month and 865 million audience impressions within 48 hours of FDA approval of Viagra were recorded as per a report in Medical Media & Marketing article.

Pfizer rallied the entire troops and encouraged everyone charged with the marketing of Viagra to push the creative envelope. The lesson is engaging and involves every team member in launching and promoting new products.

Perhaps, the most important of all lessons is how Pfizer had created a Blue Ocean for Viagra in lifestyle drugs by going beyond the boundaries of the pharmaceutical industry at the time. Pharmaceutical marketing practices traditionally revolve around functional and emotional orientation in their product offerings. Pfizer had created a lifestyle enhancement and an emotional orientation by recasting a highly stigmatized condition like impotence as erectile dysfunction. A new category was born. Pfizer created a Blue Ocean for Viagra. Viagra reigned the blue ocean space it created for itself for almost twenty years and is still managing a leading position, if not a leadership position.

Viagra has shown that when companies are willing to challenge the functional-emotional orientation of their industry, they can often create a new market space. A new blue ocean.

(Source: Adapted from articles: 1. Dominic Utton, *Viagra: The rise of erectile dysfunction drug set to be sold over-the-counter*, Express, the house of the Daily and Sunday Express, November 30, 2017, 2. Brittaney Kiefer, *Pfizer tackles erectile dysfunction taboo in the new campaign*, Campaign, April 18, 2018)

CASE

50

Mankind Pharma: Changing the Rules of the Game!

For a long time, the game of the pharmaceutical business has been running on a rulebook filled with unwritten rules. Rules such as:

1. The pyramidical structure of the business comprises factors, such as the type of therapy, doctor specialization, and drug pricing, with leading companies at the top and the majority of the firms competing fiercely in the middle.
2. Pareto's principle is at work in pharmaceutical marketing, too, with almost all the companies competing for a share of the mind of the top twenty percent of the doctors, who are specialists and are practicing in metros and tier-1 cities.
3. Specialty focus regarding therapy area and physician specialty are crucial for success.
4. There is a value at the top of the pyramid.

Changing the Rules of the Game!

The pharmaceutical industry in India, too, has been governed by these somewhat unwritten rules. At least till Mankind Pharma started its operations. Ramesh Juneja, the founder of Mankind Pharma, and his brother Rajeev Juneja, who has been heading the marketing operations since its inception in 1986, unknowingly changed the game's rules. They knew that starting a pharmaceutical company and competing with established players in Metro and Tier One cities would be next to impossible. They would not even get a second glance from the specialists and super specialists. They also knew from their experience as medical representatives and first-line sales managers in the pharmaceutical industry that the large and mid-size pharmaceutical companies focused their entire attention on top prescribers in Metro and Tier One cities (Remember the Pareto principle that 20 percent of your customers account for 80 percent of your market), and neglected general practitioners and doctors in small towns.

The Juneja brothers asked a seemingly innocent question. Everyone thinks the value is only at the top of the pyramid and focuses there. It is crowded, and start-up companies can't compete in that space. What if there is a value at the bottom of the pyramid? Can we unlock it? It is eminently possible to compete in this *no-competition zone*. They focused on the unserved and under-served market of general practitioners and all other doctors in smaller towns. The doctors in these markets forsaken by the large and mid-size pharma companies welcomed Mankind Pharma with open arms. They rewarded them with their prescriptions, making the company Number one in the number of prescriptions written in India in 2014 as per the IMS Health Report.

Rapid Growth

Coming into existence in 1986, Mankind Pharma became a corporation in 1991. The company has been highly customer-centric since its inception. The company's real growth phase started in 1995. For the next ten years or more, the company has been growing at a break-neck speed of 30 percent per year compared to the industry's 12 percent. How did Mankind Pharma achieve this extraordinary success? What is its secret sauce? Here it is in the words of Rajeev Juneja himself when he spoke to the press on different occasions: *You become creative when there is scarcity. When you have less money, no experience, no name, no background, it makes sense to tap doctors in small towns and villages. The top doctors in the metros would not have given us a second glance. The idea is to create a presence in small towns and villages and work our way up to cities.*

The Company's Secret Sauce!

The essence of the secret sauce of Mankind's strategy has been:

1. To unlock the value at the bottom of the period. The company told its medical representatives to tap as many doctors as possible and generate prescriptions. Mankind has the most extensive physician coverage in the Indian pharmaceutical industry.
2. To market their products at affordable prices. Mankind Pharma priced its products to patients at lower prices by about 30 to 40 percent, compared to the competition. The company followed Walmart's business model in marketing its products. Walmart strives to consistently lower purchase and operating costs and then pass the savings to consumers. Like Walmart, Mankind strives to keep its overheads and all other manufacturing and operating costs low and offers savings to patients. The company follows a penetrative pricing strategy. Mankind bombarded the Indian pharmaceutical market with low-priced drugs — up to 40 percent cheaper than prevailing prices, making competition sit up and take notice of this new entrant. That is why and how the company can deliver quality products at affordable prices.
3. The company has also entered the OTC (Over-the-counter) drugs and invested over Rs. 350-crore in advertising over six years to tap the OTC market and improve brand recognition. The company today has become well known with successful brands such as Manforce (Condoms), Unwanted 72 (Emergency contraceptives), and Unwanted (Home Pregnancy kits). OTC drugs account for about 8 percent of Mankind's total sales.

The strategy is working. Mankind today has become a behemoth of a company with revenues of around $930 million in 2020, and a total employee strength of about 14,000. It is noteworthy that Mankind's achievement is that its growth has been organic except for two acquisitions. The company acquired Magnet Labs in 2007 to enter the CNS (Central Nervous System) disorders and, three years later, in 2010, acquired Longifene, a UCB brand for improving appetitive in children.

What Next?

The critical question is can Mankind continue its growth spurt? Can the company maintain the high growth rate it has been used to for such a long time? Mankind seems determined to grow faster than the fastest competitor and grab market share to reach the top in the coming years. However, the company is not complacent and does not take itself for granted. The company recognizes and realizes the challenges ahead and crafts a strategy accordingly. What brought Mankind up here will not take the company to where it wants to go. It needs to change the gears. The game changer needs a new game plan. The essential elements of growth drivers of Mankind's new game plan are:

1. Increase the company's presence in the chronic therapy segment. The chronic therapy segment is growing at a higher rate of 14 percent than acute therapies, which are growing at 9.6 percent. Magnet Mankind is already making rapid strides in the segment.
2. Push the OTC segment further. It has already started contributing to the profitability of the company.
3. The domestic market alone cannot provide opportunities to grow at the current rate. Expanding into the international markets and increasing exports is vital to continue the company's frenetic pace that has become a habit. The company plans to enter the global markets in a phased and focused manner. To focus on South East Asia, Africa, CIS, and Latin America in the first phase and then graduate to the developed markets. The company plans to sell certain APIs (active

pharmaceutical ingredients) in developed markets such as the US.

4. Even in export markets, Mankind will follow its winning strategy of unlocking the value at the bottom of the pyramid. The company will also target smaller towns and cities in the export markets and offer differentiated products, not me-too products, as most of these export markets are already crowded with me-too products.
5. Move into drugs for life-threatening diseases such as cancer. The company plans to enter the oncology segment with a penetrative pricing strategy, keeping oncology drug prices 40 —60 percent cheaper than its competitors. The strategy is to approach the oncology segment with Mankind prices.
6. Foray into diagnostic space, which is going rapidly with an investment of Rs. 305-crore over four years. Pathkind is the name of the proposed diagnostic arm of the company's business. Pathkind aims to reach out to the masses in India's tier 2 and tier 3 cities to provide easily accessible diagnostic services at affordable prices. The company plans to open 12 large labs, 20 rapid response labs, and 150 collection centers in the first year in Uttarakhand states in India. The company is planning to go pan India with 1,300 collection centers and130 labs in the next five years.

Mankind is banking on higher growth from international markets in its second phase of rapid growth strategy. That is what has happened to all successful Indian Pharma majors ever since India became a signatory to GATT and a member of WTO. As a result, all the leading Indian pharmaceutical companies have started getting a significant share of their revenues from international markets. Because India currently accounts for about 5 to 6 percent of the total world Pharma market and there is a limit to what a company can exploit if it chooses to compete only in the domestic market.

Mankind is working on building the required competencies such as international marketing, formulation development, and competing in metro cities and tier-one cities. The company's impeccable track record since its inception indicates that there is every reason to believe that Mankind might as well change the game's rules for the second time!

(Source: Shabana Hussain, Mankind Pharma: Formulating a strategy to enter the big league, www.forbes.com, May 8, 2014)

In essence, Blue Ocean Strategy is the simultaneous pursuit of differentiation and low cost to open up a new market space and create new demand. It is about value innovation. It is about creating and capturing uncontested market space, thereby making the competition irrelevant. Thus, Blue Ocean Strategy is a notch above positioning and differentiation but has at its core the concept of positioning, which is differentiation.

CHAPTER

5

Framing

Frames are mental structures that shape the way of the world. If a strongly held frame doesn't fit the facts, the facts will be ignored and the frame will be kept.

— George Lakoff in his book, Don't Think of An Elephant

Framing

Erving Goffman, a Canadian-born sociologist, social psychologist, and writer, was the first to suggest the framing theory. He put forth that people interpret what is happening around their world through their primary framework. The user takes this framework as primary and takes it for granted.

In other words, Framing is about presenting information within a pre-defined interpretational frame to influence target audiences' judgment about your organization, products, or services.

Goffman also suggested two distinctions within primary frameworks—natural and social, and both help individuals interpret data so their experiences can be understood in a wider social context. Furthermore, individuals use these frameworks daily, whether they are aware of them, or not.

The US Frameworks Institute puts it succinctly when it says that Framing is the choices we make in what we say and how we say it, including what we emphasize, how and what we explain, and what we leave unsaid.

These choices matter, as they affect how people hear us, what they understand, and how they act. Word choices, too, are important as they influence people's interpretation. Therefore, the choice of your words creates a frame or theme on which to base your message. Consider these examples:

- Do you say you have an old car or a vintage car?
- Have you made mistakes or learned lessons?
- Are you heading into your twilight years or your golden years?

The Rubin Vase

In 1915, Danish psychologist Edgar Rubin developed the Rubin Vase, a good example of visual Framing. The visual effect presents the viewer with two shape interpretations, each consistent, but only one can be maintained at a given moment. For example, if you focus on the white form, you see a vase. If you focus on the black contours, you can see the outline of two faces. Rubin Vase shows us that people can perceive the same scene or scenario differently. Thus, frames can help us influence a target audience to perceive from one particular viewpoint (desired perception) instead.

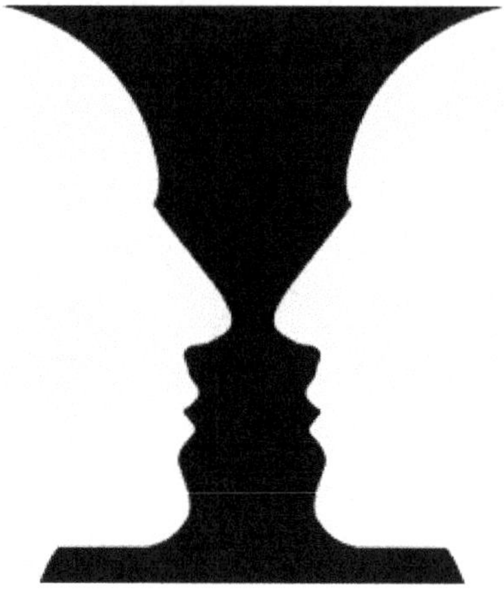

Figure 5.1 Rubin's Vase

The Science Behind Framing

We absorb new information by fitting it into the framework of something we already understand and use mental shortcuts (heuristics) to make sense of the world. These mental shortcuts rely on *frames* which are internalized concepts and values, allowing us to give meaning to new developments and information. Various elements, such as language choices, different messengers, or images, can trigger these frames and influence our decision-making.

Why Framing?

Since Framing is something that everyone does, whether conscious of it or not, two people might perceive the same scenario differently, with each person responding differently based on their perceptions. But when you frame a scenario in a certain way, everyone involved will likely look at it from that specific viewpoint. Therefore, marketers must frame their communication to their target audiences to create the desired perception in their minds.

Professor Matthew Nisbet of Northeastern University gives a strong reason why marketers should frame their messages to the target audiences when he says: *people use mental filters to make sense of incoming messages, which gives the sender (the framer) of the information enormous power to focus attention and influence how receivers will interpret the message*.

In the final analysis, Framing is about constructing, refining, and delivering messages to influence the target audiences. How the information is presented (the Frame) is crucial as it influences and changes decision-making and judgment about a product, service, or subject.

Framing and Agenda-Setting

In 1972, Maxwell McCombs and Donald Shaw proposed the Agenda-setting theory that says choosing and displaying news, editors, newsroom staff, and broadcasters play an *important part* (agenda-setting) in shaping political reality.

So is framing something like agenda setting or different? While both concepts—Framing and agenda-setting, are similar as they aim to influence a certain target audience, there is a difference. Agenda-setting tells an audience what to think, but Framing goes further and suggests how to think about an issue.

Framing in Different Contexts

Since Framing permeates our lives, Framing takes place in several contexts, with different approaches befitting each context. Falk Rehkopf, Chief Marketing Officer at UberMetrics, suggests different contexts for framing in his article, *Framing and Counter Framing in PR—Strategies, Tactics, and Tools*. Here is a summary:

- *Framing a Situation* helps with storytelling and in the context of organizational communication. Public Relations (PR) professionals use Framing to impose their version of the organization on others.
- *Framing an Attribute* is about highlighting and emphasizing certain characteristics of a product and downplaying other aspects of the same product.

- *Framing an Action* involves proposing a certain action to achieve the desired objective.
- *Framing a Risk* is essentially about influencing a person's decision-making by communicating the likelihood of a gain or loss resulting from that decision. For example, in the healthcare industry, people are more likely to agree to surgery if risks are presented in terms of survival rates (94 percent survive this operation) rather than death rates (6 percent of the people will not make it through the operation).
- *Framing a Responsibility* is when companies typically frame a responsibility in a way that allows them to take credit for successes and avoid getting blamed for failures while managing crises and in managing reputation.
- *Framing a News Story* is when organizations release news stories of new products and significant achievements in an inspiring and motivating way.

Kirk Hallahan, Professor Emeritus, Journalism and Media Communication, Colorado State University in the US, identified seven types of frames most suitable for public relations' use in his paper, *Seven Models of Framing: Implications for Public Relations*, published in the Journal of Public Relations Research on November 19, 2009. The following table presents the details.

Table 5.1 Seven Models of Framing

What is Framed?	Description	Messaging Implications
Situatons	Relationships between individuals in everyday situations	To be framed in a way that meets the expectations of participants
Attributes	-	• Emphasize aspects of causes, products and services • Product positioning cliams and price versus benefits, or quality • Example in decision-making: 60 percent success rate, or 40 percent failure rate?

Table 5.1 *Contd...*

What is Framed?	Description	Messaging Implications
Choices	Putting alternative decisions in either negative (loss), or positive (gain) terms can bias choices in situations involving uncertainty.	Greater willingness to take risks to avoid losses than taking similar risks to seek gain
Actions	In persuasive contexts, the probability that a person will act to attain a desired goal is influenced by whether alternatives are stated in positive or negative terms.	Examples: health campaigns, such as prevention of diseases, obesity, smoking, road accidents, and others
Isuues	Social problems and disputes can be explained in alternative terms by different parties who vie for their preferred definition of a problem or situation to prevail.	Defining or framing an issue builds an agenda with stakeholders, and helps gain the initiative in issues management.
Responsibity	Individuals tend to attribute cause of events to either internal, or external factors, based on levels of stability and control.	Acceptance or denial of responsibility for events, such as crisis management, corporate reputation
News	Media reports use familiar, culturally resonating themes to report on events.	Public Relations (PR) present a frame, an angle, when pitching a story to media. Journalists may frame articles to interest their largest audience segment.

(Source: Falk Rehkopf, Chief Marketing Officer, Framing and Counter Framing in PR—Strategies, Tactics and Tools, Ubermetrics, May 31, 2019)

Framing Techniques

Later, in 1996, G. T. Fairhurst and R. A. Saar suggested some framing techniques that people use in their book, *The Art of Framing: Managing the Language of Leadership*. These techniques are:

- *Metaphor*: To frame a conceptual idea through comparison to something else. Joseph Campbell, the well-known American mythologist, and writer, famously said: *If you want to change the world, change the metaphor*.
- *Stories (Myths, Legends)*: To frame a topic via narrative vividly and memorably.

- *Tradition (Rituals, Ceremonies) Cultural mores* that imbue significance in the mundane and are closely tied to artifacts.
- *Slogan, Jargon, Catchphrase*: To frame an object with a catchy phrase to make it more memorable and relatable.
- *Artifact:* Objects with intrinsic symbolic value— a visual, cultural phenomenon that holds more meaning than an object itself.
- *Contrast*: To describe an object in terms of what it is not.
- *Spin*: To present a concept in such a way as to convey a value judgment (positive or negative) that might not be immediately apparent to create an inherent bias by definition.

Framing Types

Although there are many types of Framing, almost all of them fall into the following four types:

1. Values-based frames tap into consumers' underlying values and use these to motivate certain behaviors.
2. *Financial-based* frames highlight the financial benefits of engaging in certain behaviors appealing to consumers who make decisions based on logic.
3. *Gain-based frames* focus on what consumers gain from engaging in a particular behavior.
4. *Loss-based* frames focus on what consumers lose from engaging or not engaging in a particular behavior.

Framing Effect

How you present your product and service offerings initiates a framing effect, influencing the customers' choices. The framing effect is a cognitive bias created in a person's brain based on information received. It is because people tend to react differently to the same data and information, depending on whether it is presented positively or negatively. For example, think which of these two statements are likely to evoke a positive response—*We are the third best-seller in the market*, or *Our product is one of the top three best sellers in the market*?

The editorial team at Smallbiz Technology suggests how you can use the framing effect to create messages that appeal to your customers in their blog article, *How to Implement the Framing Effect in Marketing Campaigns*, published on smallbiztechnology.com on August 1, 2022.

1. You can make your customers desire your product or service by offering them something unique when they choose your product. The ever-growing number of loyalty programs based on reward points confirm this.
2. Knowing what your customers like and don't is vital to make your value proposition that they cannot refuse.
3. Understanding the values and goals of your customers will be immensely helpful in effectively marketing your products and services based on their lifestyles. Lifestyle marketing aims to inspire, guide, and motivate customers to pursue a better way of life.
4. Always communicate the value your product can offer instead of cost.

Every product has some plusses and minuses. How you frame and present your product will influence customers' decision-making. The objective is to make customers perceive that your product offers the best value compared to the competition.

Framing in Marketing

Framing can significantly help in advertising and marketing by making your target audience feel the way you want them to in a certain way, either fear a loss or become excited about a possible gain. Since consumers respond to framing in predictable and measurable ways, it is possible to use Framing in creating your marketing messages to increase conversion rate and build customer loyalty. Liz suggests five ways to use Framing in a blog article, *Five ways to Use Framing in Your Content Marketing,* published on amplihigher.com on May 2, 2021.

1. **Loss Framing** takes advantage of predictable responses that occur when people fear loss. When faced with the choice

between a definite small loss, or an uncertain but riskier chance to avoid loss, people will choose the riskier option. For example, if a person is given $100 and has to choose whether to lose $50 or flip a coin where the consequences were losing or keeping the entire $100, most people would select the coin flip. While loss framing seems illogical, this paradoxical response is due to the risk aversion in human nature. Surprisingly, marketers use loss framing more often than gain framing. The most common examples of this are the ubiquitous offer signs in stores worldwide saying—*Limited-time Offer* and Last *Chance—Don't Miss out*! Loss framing is very popular because most people fear a loss more than they desire a gain.

2. **Gain Framing** is where certainty wins. Gain framing highlights what the customer stands to attain by taking action. It allows you to emphasize the positive aspects of your products, services, or company and helps you build your brand's reputation, increasing perceived value and trustworthiness. Customers choose the safest option when faced with a definite small gain or a chance at a larger gain. So gain framing is perfect for situations where the outcome is certain, whereas loss framing is better for uncertain conditions.
3. **Hyperbolic Discounting**: People typically choose the immediate reward when given the option between a small, immediate reward and a larger one that requires waiting. Hyperbolic discounting incentivizes people to act immediately, using the time to increase perceived value. Common examples of hyperbolic discounting are the reward points offered by credit card companies and frequent-flyer programs airlines. The rewards, such as 100 points, typically seem more than their actual value and may equal only about $5.
4. **Statistical Framing**: Statistics and ratios are often used in advertising and marketing because they make your message seem more authentic and trustworthy regardless of whether you use them in a positive (our product is 80 percent effective) or negative (competitor's product fails 1 out of 5 times) frame. Use statistical Framing to establish the credibility and superiority of your products.

5. **Emotional Framing**: Words are powerful triggers of emotion. That is why the choice of words is very important in Emotional Framing. For example, framing a person's cancer situation as a journey rather than a battle is more likely to encourage coping. On the contrary, a battle frame (metaphor) evokes negative emotions, such as a lack of recovery as a defeat and potentially a personal failure.

Whatever your marketing goals are, you will always use Framing to communicate your message. In addition, understanding the different framing concepts will help you elicit the reactions and responses you want from your target audience. Therefore, mastering framing techniques is vital for making marketing communications more effective and memorable.

Frame of Reference

Creating a frame of reference is the starting point of marketing a new product or service. It helps customers identify a new product and its category so they can compare and evaluate the relative benefits of products in the category. Thus, the *Frame of Reference* concept clarifies the value proposition of your product and positions it within the market.

After establishing a frame of reference for the brand, the next step is to communicate the superiority of your product over its competitors' products. The two ways to do this are by comparing your products on—points of parity and points of difference.

You should dwell on points of parity only if your product offers your customers some benefits that your competitors cannot offer.

After proving the product's superiority over points of parity, it is time to highlight the points of difference that only your product can offer and communicate its differential advantage.

Getting Your Framing Right

The three most important points you must remember when formulating your framing strategies are:

1. Focus on the core objective of your message, be it regarding your product or company.
2. Focus on your most important target audience segment. While it is tempting to appeal to all customer segments simultaneously, it is impossible. Remember the adage? When you stand for everything, you stand for nothing.
3. Stick to the core and provide only the compelling evidence, reinforcing the Framing.

The following are some examples of pharmaceutical companies that used Framing to craft their messages to physicians to promote their brands.

Framing Messages in Pharma Marketing: Some Examples

- Cialis-the Erectile Dysfunction drug changed the reference point from sex to romance.
- Fosamax, the osteoporosis drug, touched the emotional chords of customers and consumers with its *Emotional Framing*—freedom from fractures!
- Bayer in India changed the Frame of reference with its Alert theme for its anti-allergic Incidal as a daytime antihistamine.
- Roche changed the frame of reference visually to its injectable antibiotic brand, Rocephin. While all other injectable products used images of scary, open, infected wounds and blown-up microscopic pathogens in their promotional literature and visual aids, the Rocephin brand management team followed a different route by showing the image of an apple, denoting the simple yet folksy adage that an apple a day keeps the doctor away. They reframed the kill power of the antibacterial drug (the positioning of other injectable antibiotics at the time) to wellness and rapid recovery from infections.
- Ultradol —reframed customer perception by communicating its lower gastrointestinal side effects and convenience of a once-daily dosage and positioned it as a safer analgesic.
- Capoten of BMS developed captopril for severe hypertension, and MSD developed its ACE inhibitor, Vasotec, at lower doses for mild to moderate hypertension.

- Merck changed the reference point of diabetes treatment from sugar control to the HbA1c test standard in promoting its Januvia and Janumet brands for treating diabetes.

The following case shows how Johnson & Johnson changed the frame of reference in treating peptic ulcers with Pepcid's launch strategy in the UK.

CASE

51

Pepcid's Positioning Strategy for UK Launch Helps the Brand to Fight the Mighty Zantac Effectively!

In 1987, Johnson & Johnson launched its antiulcerant drug, Pepcid (famotidine), an H2 antagonist, in the UK when Zantac was ruling the antiulcerant market. And in 1988, Glaxo's (GlaxoSmithKline, now) Zantac (ranitidine) became the world's best-selling prescription drug.

Competing head-on with a firmly entrenched brand like Zantac did not seem possible. So, Johnson & Johnson had to find a differential advantage, and they found one. That was about blocking nocturnal acid in patients with peptic ulcers. Leading gastroenterologists say that blocking nocturnal acid is the key to peptic ulcer therapy. Pepcid has superior efficacy in blocking nocturnal acid levels than Zantac. Johnson & Johnson found its secret sauce and positioned it as *the first acid regulator designed for once-a-night use*.

Here's how Johnson & Johnson communicated the differential advantage of Pepcid to HCPs (Healthcare Professionals):

During the day, the patient needs normal gastric acid for natural digestion and protection against unwanted intestinal bacteria.

Pepcid (famotidine) is the new H2 receptor antagonist that works the way you want an acid suppressant to work. Pepcid is designed to stop acid at night when your patients don't need it, and not during the day when they do. Clinical tests show that Pepcid is superior to Zantac (ranitidine) in reducing nighttime gastric acid. During the nighttime, Pepcid reduced gastric acid by 16 percent below the levels achieved by Zantac. Yet during daytime hours, Pepcid and Zantac were equivalent.

Pepcid achieved healing within 4 to 8 weeks in almost all cases of peptic ulcers.

That's the new Pepcid. A single once-a-night 40 mg tablet that promotes rapid pain relief and ulcer healing by blocking nocturnal acid.

And for the patient, Pepcid comes in convenient 28-day calendar packs.

Review and Test Your Messages

Reviewing and testing your messages to detect any confusing words or phrases is important. Test among employees from different areas of your organization if it is an internal message. If it is an external message, test it among a representative sample of the target audience. The key questions to ask while reviewing messages are:

- Does this message make sense?
- How does this message make you feel?
- What do you think this message is asking you to do? What is the call for action?
- Who do you think this message will resonate with?
- What would you change about this message to make it speak directly to you?
- Which message do you think will resonate most? Why?

CHAPTER

6

Brand Positioning in The Digital Age

How do we get found in Search Engines? How do we get people to talk about us on Social? We better be interesting and helpful, and we better do that on a consistent basis.

—Joe Pulizzi, A top Content Marketing Authority and founder of the Content Marketing Institute

Brand Positioning in The Digital Age

The fourth industrial revolution we are witnessing is unlike any other, with 90 percent of data produced in the last two years and more than 26 billion smart devices in circulation.

Paradoxical as it may seem, despite the giant technological strides we have made in automation, artificial intelligence, and machine learning, the essence of human connection—eye contact, personal touch, empathy—remain irreplaceable by technology according to recent research by Deloitte, a global management consultancy major.

The Human Experience Quotient

Amelia Dunlop, Ashley Reichheld, Jannine Zucker, Maggie Gross, Christine Kang, and Laura Martin at Deloitte Digital developed an algorithm, the human experience quotient, that indicates where an organization is along the journey to elevate the human experience. They distilled their learnings in an article, *What did we learn from measuring human values*, published in their blog on Deloitte Digital. Understanding the human experience quotient helps companies align with the values of their customers, workers, and partners. They have uncovered five important core human tenets in elevating the human experience.

1. Be obsessed by all things human.
2. Proactively deliver on human needs.
3. Execute with humanity
4. Be authentic.
5. Change the world.

Brands in the Digital Age: Seven Trends

Customers expect brands to treat them like humans, not merely as transactions, and to embody human qualities. *Deloitte's first Global Marketing Trends report* identifies seven marketing trends that indicate a human-first philosophy. These seven trends are:

1. **Purpose:** A purpose-driven brand helps connect with customers on a deeper level and build enduring relationships,

making it a core differentiator. As Richard Branson, the iconoclastic entrepreneur and founder of the Virgin Group, says: *The brands that will thrive in the coming year are the ones that have a purpose beyond profit*. Customers prefer purpose-driven brands. Over 80 percent of customers say when they buy a product from a purpose-driven company, they feel they are taking some part in making a positive impact. Above all, companies that lead with purpose and build around it can achieve continued loyalty, consistency, and relevance in consumers' lives.

2. **Human Experience:** Even though technology can replicate human behavior and gestures through automation and artificial intelligence, it cannot replace the essentials of human connection— eye contact, personal touch, and empathy. Empathy is walking in another person's shoes. Metaphorically speaking, it is an effort to grasp their point of view emotionally. Empathy enables you to better design your products and services for the human experience as you understand your stakeholders find meaning and belonging in products and services.
3. **Fusion:** Fusion is about the convergence of ecosystems erasing the traditional boundaries between industries. For example, non-traditional players—big tech companies, such as Amazon, Apple, Alphabet, Microsoft, and some tech startup companies are entering the healthcare space with innovative technologies to improve customer experiences in their healthcare journeys. Fusion amplifies the marketing myopia concept of expanding a brand's perspective proposed by Levitt over sixty-plus years ago. It means looking beyond industry boundaries, finding new ways to serve customer needs, and partnering with former competitors.
4. **Trust:** The digital era makes trust a complex issue accompanied by many existential threats, including external cyber threats and unethical internal data misuse. Companies must build a structure that systemically builds trust by protecting customer data from these. They should understand that data belongs to customers, and brands are the stewards

of this customer asset. They must be transparent and upfront in their intentions and actions.

5. **Participation:** Marketers increasingly realize that two-way engagement across all stages of the consumer journey and the product lifecycle is crucial to successful brand building. In the digital age, where consumers are becoming the brand *media*, participating in developing products and services, involving them is the only way to convert consumers into brand advocates.
6. **Talent:** The importance of nurturing and developing talent can never be overemphasized. Companies must understand how to acquire and grow talent and create an environment for good employee experience where talent can thrive. Because people with positive experiences only can create and improve customer experiences.
7. **Agility:** The digital age makes it mandatory for organizations to adopt, learn, and implement agile practices because an agile mindset enables them to keep up with the speed of culture, conversation, and digitization that has become the norm in today's digital world.

Brand Positioning in the Digital Age

Even in the digital age, the fundamentals of brand positioning remain the same. It is the foundation for building a strong brand, requiring a product or service concept and a targeted group of consumers. The positioning then articulates what the company wants consumers to think about the brand. It does so by framing the brand as a familiar way of achieving a goal and highlighting a basis of superiority relative to other alternatives in the frame.

While a brand typically can be positioned in more than one way, it is important to select the most compelling positioning for the target, provide a sizable market, and be defensible overtime against the competition.

The brand positioning statement, too, in today's hyper-connected world, remains unchanged. A formal positioning statement continues to include in the digital age four elements: a target, a frame of reference, a point of difference, and a reason to believe. The brand positioning statement is an internal document to align all consumer-facing decisions related to the brand, such as decisions about elements of brand design, touchpoints, messaging, and others. Its main objective is to keep everyone concerned with brand-building in the organization on the same page. In addition, the brand positioning strategy must ensure alignment of frame of reference, point of difference, and reason to believe in making it effective and maximizing demand.

What is changing? Emphasis on brand purpose. The importance of purpose in brand building is growing, with over 1.8 billion millennials five times more likely to stay with a company with a strong connection to its purpose than non-millennials, who are only about two times more likely to stay. Therefore it is important to include the brand purpose— its *raison d'être* in your brand positioning statement and, more importantly, to live it!

Another change in the digital age is how customers engage with brands with the onset of digital platforms. Today, marketers must provide a holistic brand experience to create a sustainable differential advantage.

Holistic marketing is about ensuring all parts and employees of the organization understand the brand, and their role in enhancing the brand experience.

In today's digital environment, it is possible to personalize brand engagement to meet consumer needs, with data and analytics, insights, and content marketing research done in real-time reinforcing conventional brand strategies.

Positioning for Patients

Although patient centricity is a familiar buzzword in the pharmaceutical industry today, most pharma companies still largely target and focus prescribers. But, of course, HCPs (Healthcare Professionals) are a very important target audience for pharma as they make the prescribing decisions on behalf of the patient— the end user. As a result, the brand positioning statement primarily highlights the benefits their products offer to physicians. However, patients who have been passive recipients of healthcare are increasingly taking a more active role in their healthcare decision-making today. Also, physicians' exclusive role in prescribing decisions is slowly diluting, with other stakeholders becoming more active than before.

Many experts echo the increasing participation of patients in managing their health. Here are some experts' opinions:

- Bertalan Mesko, a medical futurist and author, said: *Healthcare will be driven much more by consumers than physicians, with patients increasingly coming to their doctors with more information, parameters they measured at home, and an informed opinion about how they should be treated*.
- Dan Goldsmith, the chief strategy officer of Veeva Systems, a cloud-based life-science business-solutions company, predicts: *In the next three to five years, instead of patients being informed and more interested, they will be actively designing the therapeutic and treatment approaches for themselves with their physicians*.

And yet, most pharma companies focus their brand positioning on benefits to the physician. However, one pharma company started positioning its prescription drug brand for the patient. The following case presents the details.

CASE

52

How Eli Lilly Positioned its Prescription Drug Brand for the Patient and Won?!

One global pharma major, Eli Lilly & Company, started a patient-centric positioning for their Cialis (tadalafil), a third-in-class erectile dysfunction drug, in 2003, much before patient-centricity became a buzzword.

Pfizer's Viagra (sildenafil) was the brand leader in the erectile dysfunction market, with a dominant share of about seventy percent in 2003. Viagra created the Erectile dysfunction market.

Cialis was not only a late entrant to the market but also had a slower onset of action and longer duration of action. Physicians thought that this was a disadvantage, while patients felt otherwise. They associated Cialis with intimacy and romance and not just sex. The marketing team listened to the patients and changed the frame of reference for Cialis in treating erectile dysfunction accordingly, making it a primary point of differentiation. They built their marketing campaigns around it. Without a doubt, Lilly's patient-centric positioning made Cialis a big success!

(Source: Jeanne Ryan, Principal, Marketing at ZS Associates, *Brand Positioning in Pharma: Where's the Patient?* ZS Associates, zs.com)

Jeanne Ryan, Principal, Marketing at ZS Associates, suggests three key steps to developing a patient-centric approach to brand positioning in her article, *Brand Positioning in Pharma: Where's the Patient,* published in ZS Associates blog, zs.com.

1. Develop your brand positioning with the patient at the center, focusing on meaningful benefits for the patient, which all stakeholders care about.
2. Explore new territories with patients. Take time and listen to patients and understand the core benefits to the patient and how these benefits impact patients' lives. Innovative research approaches, such as mobile ethnographies and co-creation sessions, can help develop a deeper understanding of patient needs.
3. Link the positioning to customer-specific benefits and messaging. While focusing on the patient for brand positioning, you must communicate the resulting benefit to other stakeholders, such as HCPs, because when the patient benefits, they also benefit. For example, if your drug is the easiest to use for patients, focusing your message on how it can reduce HCPs' concerns about compliance can resonate with the physicians. Highlighting these physician-oriented benefits and elements like the pharmaceutical company's reputation can be important differentiating factors where there is little or no difference between the two products regarding product attributes and functional benefits.

Finally, the impact on the patient's life should be the focus of your brand positioning as it is the patient experiencing the symptoms, the symptom relief, the side effects, and a better or worsening prognosis. It is the way to win the customers' hearts and minds and improve patient outcomes.

Epilogue
Position, or Perish!

Every day in Africa, a gazelle wakes up knowing he must outrun the fastest lion or perish. At the same time, a lion stirs and stretches, knowing he must outrun the fastest gazelle or starve. It's no different for the human race. Whether you consider yourself a gazelle, or a lion, you have to run faster than others to survive.

— *Mohammed bin Rashid Al Maktoum*

Position, or Perish!

Developing a unique and compelling positioning is your only weapon to fight and defend against the competition in today's hyper-competitive and over-communicated marketplace.

Positioning strategy is crucial for building your brands and guiding a wide range of strategic decisions, such as brand identity, messaging, service culture, strategic partnerships, and many others.

The Four *Ps* to Four *E s*

Introduced in the 1940s by McCarthy, the four 'P' s have come a long way and are still important. However, the current marketing environment, which has shifted from a manufacturing mindset and product orientation to a customer-focused mindset and customer orientation dictates and demands a change. The four 'E' framework, suggested by Laura Bates and Karen McStern, partners at Brand Verve, a Strategic branding consulting firm, in their article, *Position or Perish: Positioning Your Brand to Thrive*, published in IFA (International Franchise Association) blog on December 4, 2017, is more relevant today. Here are the four Es—Experience, Economics, Engagement, and Employees.

1. **Experience**: In the traditional marketing model, the focus has been on functions, specifications, formulas, and technological superiorities. While these are still important today, the focus is shifting to customer experience. With digital and technological advancements, several industries have been delivering seamless customer experiences with their products and services to consumers across all touchpoints of their journey. As a result, consumers, having been used to those experiences, began expecting the same even from healthcare, including pharmaceuticals. Therefore, pharma companies must provide superior, differentiated experiences across all touchpoints to consumers and customers on their journeys. And experiences are not just attributes and benefits of products and services but are multi-sensory, physical, virtual, and

immersive. It is only possible when you go omnichannel in marketing.

2. **Economics:** Pricing in the traditional marketing model involves establishing the right price for the product. The right price is still important. However, the focus is shifting to value not only for the end user but for payers, too, in terms of successful outcomes. Many new value-based pricing models, and pay-for-performance are being studied to determine the optimal economic value.
3. **Engagement:** In the traditional marketing model, Promotion relied heavily on persuasively pushing promotional messages about product superiority and benefits to physicians. However, persuasion and pushing promotional messages are not enough today. Engagement is essential. We must understand consumers' needs deeply, earn their trust and engage them beyond the typical purchase cycle. Pharma can learn from Domino's Pizza which has evolved and innovated by listening to customers and acting on the customer feedback re-engineered their whole business, co-creating with customer inputs.
4. **Employees**: How can you get the best out of your employees so they can deliver superior customer experiences? Only by empowering them to act as ambassadors of our brands. We must train them to be experts and empathetic, responsive, and resourceful. Pharma can learn from Southwest Airlines, which actively seeks to recruit people with a *warrior spirit, a servant's heart, and a fun-loving attitude*.

Review Your Positioning

You must review and refine your positioning strategy as the market environment and consumer needs constantly change. Furthermore, successful positioning is not achieved overnight but evolves. Therefore, you should sculpt your positioning over time to build your brand into a living, breathing part of your customers' lives.

Here are some key questions for reviewing your positioning strategy.

- Does your brand's perception continue to be consistent with customers' deeper needs? Is it the same as you have planned?
- Are your core customers aging out of the market?
- If they are, what about new customers and their deeper needs? Does your brand meet those and resonate with them?
- What about your brand's market share? Are you gaining or losing?
- Are your competitors growing faster than you? Are there any new competitors entering your space?
- What about your brand's growth rate? Are you growing faster than the market and competition?
- How relevant is your brand to today's customers? Is it losing relevance?

You can determine whether you should refine your positioning, reposition your brand, or launch a new one to disrupt the market.

You must constantly tend your brands to stay relevant. Positioning is not a one time exercise but needs to be continually assessed and fine-tuned because customers' needs are not constant but change. Competitors do not stand still, and new industries continuously disrupt the market and alter the game.

The message is loud and clear. Keep your positioning fresh and relevant, or your brand and organization may perish.

References

1. Al Ries and Jack Trout, *Positioning: The Battle for Your Mind*, Warner books, New York, 1982
2. Jack Trout with Steve Rivkin, *Repositioning: Marketing in An Era of Competition, Change, and Crisis*, McGraw Hill Publishing,
3. Marcel Corstjens, *Marketing Strategy in the Pharmaceutical Industry*, Chapman & Hall, New York, 1991
4. Michael J. Barratt, Donald E. Frail, *Drug Repositioning: Bringing New Life to Shelved Assets and Existing Drugs*, Wiley Publication, Kindle Edition, 2012
5. Jagadish N. Seth, The Self-Destructive Habits of Good Companies And How To Break Them, Wharton School Publishing, 2007
6. Vince Parry, President of 'Y' Brand, *Branding A Disease*, Pharmaceutical Executive, October 15, 2007, https://www.pharmexec.com/view/branding-disease
7. Ulli Appelbaum, *The Brand Positioning Workbook: A Simple How-to-Guide to More Compelling Brand Positionings, Faster,* Kindle Edition, 2022
8. Markus Saba & Hilary Gentile, *Brand Plan Rx: The Marketers Guide to Building A Thriving Health and Wellness Brand*, BrightWing Media, Kindle Edition, 2022
9. Marco De Veglia, *Brand Positioning Formula: The Practical Step-by-Step Guide to Use Brand Positioning in Your Marketing*, Kindle Edition, 2018
10. April Dunford, *Obviously Awesome: How to Nail Product Positioning So Customers Get It, Buy it, Love It*, Bright Wing Books, Kindle Edition, 2019
11. Professor Brian D. Smith, *Brand Therapy: 15 Techniques for Creating Brand Strategy in Pharma and Medtech*, Practical Inspiration Publishing, Kindle Edition, 2018
12. Richard D. Czerniawski and Michael W. Maloney, *Competitive Positioning: Best Practices for Creating Brand Loyalty*, Hudson House Publishing, Kindle Edition, 2010
13. Mike Rea, *Pharmaceutical Positioning*, IDEA Pharma, Kindle Edition, 2020

14. Beata Borucka, SWOT & SO WHAT: Exceptional Practical Guide to Every Marketer, Exertus Group Limited, Kindle Edition, 2018
15. George Lakoff, Don't Think of An Elephant: Know Your Values and Frame the Debate, Chelsea Green Publishing, Tenth Anniversary Edition, 2014
16. Stan Bernard, President, Bernard Associates, *Product Positioning 2.0*, Pharmaceutical Executive, February 1, 2014, https://www.pharmexec.com/view/product-positioning-20
17. Adam Williams, *How to Effectively Use Horizontal Brand Positioning to Beat Your Competitors*, speakwithadam.com, December 9, 2014, http://www.speakwithadam.com/effectively-use-horizontal-brand-positioning-beat-competitors/
18. Envoy, *10 Reasons to Reposition Your Brand*, weareenvoymedium.com, October 23, 2018, https://weareenvoy.medium.com/10-reasons-to-reposition-your-brand-2c7e8beb954f
19. *5 Keys to Positioning Pharmaceutical Products*, The Marchitect, January 26, 2011, https://mytubefacetwitter.wordpress.com/2011/01/26/5-keys-to-positioning-pharmaceutical-products
20. Scot Seidewitz, *The Last Thing You Should Think About When Positioning A New Drug (Hint: It's the Drug)*, The Seidewitz Group, September 28, 2017 https://www.seidewitzgroup.com/blog/positioning-a-new-drug-the-last-thing-you-should-think-about-is-your-drug
21. Jean-Pierre Jourdan, Ronan Bureau, Christophe Rochais, Patrick Dailemagne, *Drug Repositioning: A Brief Overview*, Journal of Pharmacy and Pharmacology / Volume 72, Issue 9, p. 1145—1151, Wiley Online Library, https://onlinelibrary.wiley.com/doi/full/10.1111/jphp.13273
22. Miner J, Hoffhines A, *The discovery of aspirin's antithrombotic effects*. Tex Heart Inst J. 2007;34(2):179-86. PMID: 17622365; PMCID: PMC1894700, https://pubmed.ncbi.nlm.nih.gov/?term=Hoffhines%20A%5BAuthor%5D

23. Mithun Rudrapal, Shubham J. Khairnar and Anil G. Jadhav, *Drug Repurposing (DR): An Emerging Approach in Drug Discovery*, Intechopen, July 13, 2020, https://www.intechopen.com/chapters/72744
24. Dinsa Sachan, *The Thalidomide Story Explained*, Down To Earth, April 30, 2010, https://www.downtoearth.org.in/news/the-thalidomide-story-explained-1028
25. Medically Reviewed by Kristin Hall, FNP, Written by Editorial Team at HIMS (Health Management Information System), Revatio Vs. Viagra: What's the Difference? HIMS, September 2, 2020, https://www.forhims.com/blog/revatio-vs-viagra-whats-difference
26. Christoph Abels, Micheal Soeberdt, Can We Teach Old Drugs New Tricks— Repurposing of Neuropharmacological drugs For Inflammatory Skin Diseases., June 7, 2019Experimental Dermatology/Volume 28, Issue 9/ p.1002-1009, Wiley Online Library, https://onlinelibrary.wiley.com/doi/full/10.1111/exd.13987
27. John Crudele, Hair Growth Drug Seen As A Wonder For Upjohn, The New York Times, May 28, 1985, https://www.nytimes.com/1985/05/28/business/hair-growth-drug-seen-as-a-wonder-for-upjohn.html
28. The Accidental Discovery of Minoxidil And Other Medicines, Hims, https://www.forhims.co.uk/blog/minoxidil-accidental-discovery
29. Brainiac, How Claude Hopkins Manipulated the World to Use Toothpaste—Pepsodent Hopkin's History, kickstartersidehustle.com, https://kickstartsidehustle.com/how-claude-hopkins-manipulated-the-world-to-use-toothpaste-pepsodent-history/
30. Falk Rehkopf, Chief Marketing Officer, Framing and Counter Framing in PR—Strategies, Tactics and Tools, Ubermetrics, May 31, 2019, https://www.ubermetrics-technologies.com/blog/framing-and-counter-framing-in-communications-strategies-tactics/

31. Paul Boyce, Framing Effect Definition, BoyceWire, February 8, 2021, https://boycewire.com/framing-effect-definition-and-examples/
32. Kate Schoen, *Priming VS. Framing in Marketing*, Halcon Marketing, July 5, 2021, https://www.halconmarketing.com/post/priming-vs-framing-in-marketing
33. Indeed Editorial Team, *What is Message Framing? (With Types and Tips for Use)*, indeed.com, May 19, 2022, https://www.indeed.com/career-advice/career-development/message-framing
34. *Framing Theory*, Mass Communication Theory, https://masscommtheory.com/theory-overviews/framing-theory/
35. Tréa Lavery, Editorial Assistant, *Definition: Framing Effec*t, techtarget.com, Last Updated in February 2017, https://www.techtarget.com/whatis/definition/framing-effect
36. Gerald Hanks, *Framing Examples in Advertising*, CHRON, March 8, 2019, https://smallbusiness.chron.com/examples-hyperbole-advertising-66083.html
37. Kim Harrison, *Frame Your Key Messages for Best Results*, Cutting Edge PR, June 1, 2020, https://cuttingedgepr.com/frame-your-key-messages-for-best-results/
38. Dr. Leandro Herrero, *Framing of Messages is Essential for Strong Leadership*, Cutting Edge PR, October, 17, 2020, https://cuttingedgepr.com/framing-of-messages-is-essential-for-strong-leadership/
39. Jon Persson, Brand Identity Designer, *Are You Framing Your Brand Properly*, CultMethod, https://cultmethod.com/articles/framing/
40. Alex Moskov, 12 Powerful Framing Dialogues: Know What to Say, Close More Deals, Red Bear Negotiation, November 2, 2021, https://www.redbearnegotiation.com/test/concede-according-to-plan-to-conquer-negotiations-0
41. Abhimanyu Shekhawat, The Concept of Framing, LinkedIn Blog, February 10, 2016, https://www.linkedin.com/pulse/concept-framing-abhimanyu-shekhawat/

42. Colin Finkle, *Framing Effect in Marketing and Advertising*, Brand Marketing Blog, August 16, 2019, https://brandmarketingblog.com/articles/branding-how-to/framing-effect-in-marketing-and-advertising/
43. Kitty Shui, *Framing in Marketing: Back to Basics*, Digital Academy, https://www.digitalalchemy.global/framing-in-marketin/
44. Clara Franco, *Framing Theory in Marketing*, LinkedIn Blog, December 1, 2021, https://www.linkedin.com/pulse/framing-theory-marketing-carla-franco/
45. Surabhi Kedia, *5 Types of Framing Effects in Marketing*, Marketing Media, November 20, 2020, https://www.marketingmind.in/5-types-of-framing-effects-in-marketing/
46. Ciaran John, *What is Frame of Reference in Marketing?* CHRON Newsletters, Updated March 12, 2019, https://smallbusiness.chron.com/frame-reference-marketing-31287.html
47. David Aaker, Vice Chairman, *3 Ways to Re-frame Your Category*, Prophet Blog, https://www.prophet.com/2014/04/189-3-ways-to-re-frame-your-category-and-win/
48. Liz, *5 Ways to Use Framing in Your Content Marketing*, AMPLIHIGHER, May 2, 2021, https://amplihigher.com/5-ways-to-use-framing-in-your-content-marketing/
49. S. Ramesh Kumar, *Brand Fallibility in the Digital Age*, ET Brand Equity, June 21, 2021, https://brandequity.economictimes.indiatimes.com/news/marketing/brand-fallibility-in-the-digital-age/83705386
50. S. Ramesh Kumar, and S. Swaminathan, *Holistic Brand Experience in the Digital Age*, ET Brand Equity, October 30, 2020, https://brandequity.economictimes.indiatimes.com/news/marketing/holistic-brand-experience-in-the-digital-age/78934842
51. Michael Georgiou, *How And Why to Build Brand Authenticity*, Forbes, March 15, 2021, https://brandequity.economictimes.indiatimes.com/news/marketing/holistic-brand-experience-in-the-digital-age/78934842

52. Amelia Dunlop, Ashley Reichheld, Jannine Zucker, Maggie Gross, Christine Kang, and Laura Martin, *We're Only Human: Exploring and Quantifying the Human Experience*, Deloitte Digital, August 7, 2019, https://www.deloittedigital.com/us/en/blog-list/2019/we-re-only-human—exploring-and-quantifying-the-human-experience.html
53. Jeanne Ryan, *Brand Positioning in Pharma: Where's the Patient*? ZS Associates, https://www.zs.com/insights/brand-positioning-in-pharma-where-is-the-patient
54. Yaron Landow, *A Brand Positioning Nightmare*, Pharmaceutical Executive, June 1, 2012, https://www.pharmexec.com/view/brand-positioning-nightmare
55. Laura Bates and Karen McSteen, *Position or Perish: Positioning Your Brand to Thrive*, IFA: International Franchise Association, December 4, 2017, https://www.franchise.org/franchise-information/marketing/position-or-perish-positioning-your-brand-to-thrive
56. Lea Prevel Katsanis, Erica Leonard, *The Dimensions of Prescription Drug Brand Personality as Identified by Consumers*, Journal of Consumer Marketing, January 2013, 30 (7): 583-596, https://www.researchgate.net/publication/263083423_The_dimensions_of_prescription_drug_brand_personality_as_identified_by_consumers
57. Kevin Lane Keller, Brian Sternthal, and Alice M. Tybout, *Three Questions You Need to Ask About Your Brand*, Harvard Business Review, September 2002, https://hbr.org/2002/09/three-questions-you-need-to-ask-about-your-brand
58. *David Aaker, Points of Parity and Consumer's Brand Preference*, Prophet Blog, https://hbr.org/2002/09/three-questions-you-need-to-ask-about-your-brand
59. Coralyn Loomis, *Brand Personification: The Ultimate Way to Get to Know Your Brand*, Marketing Profs, https://www.marketingprofs.com/articles/2016/29950/brand-personification-the-ultimate-way-to-get-to-know-your-brand
60. Leonard Lerer, *Pharmaceutical Marketing Segmentation in the Age of the Internet*, International Journal of Medical Marketing, January 2002, https://www.researchgate.net/publication/233498277_Pharmaceutical_Marketing_Segmentation_in_the_Age_of_the_Internet

61. Gardiner Harris, *After Five Years, Rivals Emerge to Give Viagra a Fight*, The New York Times, August 21, 2003, https://www.nytimes.com/2003/08/21/business/after-5-years-rivals-emerge-ready-to-give-viagra-a-fight.html

62. Cialis: *Building More Loving Relationships in Commerce*, What If! Part of Accenture, https://whatifinnovation.com/case_studies/cialis/

63. *Azithromycin: A World Best-Selling Antibiotic*, WIPO (World Intellectual Property Organization), https://www.wipo.int/ipadvantage/en/details.jsp?id=906

64. *It took a Brilliant Marketing Campaign to Create the Best-Selling Drug of All Time*, businessinsider.com, December 28, 2011

65. Christopher Bowe, *Say Farewell to Lipitor, But Don't Forget its Lessons*, Harvard Business Review, November 18, 2011, https://hbr.org/2011/11/say-farewell-to-lipitor-but-do

66. Paul Rodgers, *The House that Zantac Built: Glaxo Pins its Hopes on a New High-tech Research Center in Stevenage*, February 5, 1995, Independent, https://www.independent.co.uk/news/business/the-house-that-zantac-built-1571538.html

67. Carl Elliot, *How to Brand A Disease—And Sell A Cure*, CNN Special, October 2010, http://edition.cnn.com/2010/OPINION/10/11/elliott.branding.disease/index.html

68. Jacqueline Mumford, *From SWOT to "So What?": A New Method For Analyzing Outcomes*, Lassonde Entrepreneur Institute, December 24, 2017, https://lassonde.utah.edu/from-swot-to-so-what-a-new-method-for-analyzing-outcomes/

69. Margaret L. Eaton, Mark Xu, *Developing and Marketing a Blockbuster Drug: Lessons from Eli Lilly's Experience with Prozac*, Harvard Business Publishing Education, February 25, 2006. https://hbsp.harvard.edu/product/BME6-PDF-ENG

70. Jeremy Laurance, *Health Check: Science Created Prozac but Marketing Made it Sing*, Independent, February 2, 1999, https://www.independent.co.uk/arts-entertainment/health-check-science-created-prozac-but-marketing-made-it-sing-1068214.html

Index

E

F

G

H

I

J

S

T

U

V

X

Z

ABOUT THE AUTHOR

Subba Rao Chaganti has a masters in business administration and over fifty-five years of experience in pharmaceutical marketing covering the whole gamut and all facets of the industry from selling to sales management, product management to heading the total marketing activity. His experience covers domestic and international marketing, and also Indian and multinational sectors.

He also taught for a few years a course on Advertising and Brand Management at Gitam Institute of Foreign Trade (now part of Gitam University) at Visakhapatnam as an adjunct professor and also taught a course on Marketing at Jawaharlal Nehru Technological University (JNTU), Hyderabad as a visiting faculty.

He lives in Hyderabad and can be reached at subbarao.chaganti@gmail.com

Here is a list of his publications:

Books Published:

1. Pharmaceutical marketing in India: Concepts, Cases, Strategy
2. Game Plans for Post-Gatt Era: Action Agenda of Indian Pharmaceutical Industry
3. Compete or Forfeit: Strategies for Sustainable Competitive Advantage in Pharma Product Patents Era
4. Pharmaceutical Marketing in India for Today and Tomorrow - 25th Anniversary Edition
5. Bullseyes and Blunders: Lessons from 100 Cases in Pharma Marketing
6. Digital Pharma Marketing Playbook: Winning With the New Rules of Engagement
7. Cracking the Generics Code: Your Single-Source Success Manual for Winning in Multi-Source Product Markets
8. Reimagine Pharma Marketing: Make It Future-Proof!

CPSIA information can be obtained
at www.ICGtesting.com
Printed in the USA
LVHW061320070123
736514LV00026B/98

9 789395 039512